4 Hands Are Better Than 2

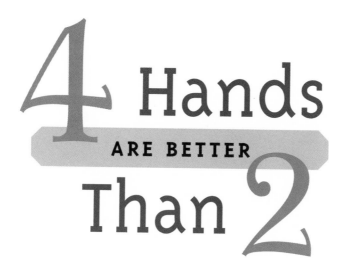

4 Hands ARE BETTER Than 2

A Guide for Original Tandem Massage

TERRI TREMPER, NCTMB
and TAMMI TREMPER, NCTMB

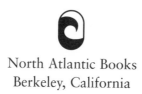

North Atlantic Books
Berkeley, California

Published by
North Atlantic Books
P.O. Box 12327
Berkeley, California 94712

Cover and book design by Suzanne Albertson
Printed in the United States of America

Distributed to the book trade by Publishers Group West

4 Hands Are Better Than 2: A Guide for Original Tandem Massage is sponsored by the Society for the Study of Native Arts and Sciences, a nonprofit educational corporation whose goals are to develop an educational and crosscultural perspective linking various scientific, social, and artistic fields; to nurture a holistic view of arts, sciences, humanities, and healing; and to publish and distribute literature on the relationship of mind, body, and nature.

North Atlantic Books' publications are available through most bookstores. For further information, call 800-337-2665 or visit our website at www.northatlanticbooks.com.

Substantial discounts on bulk quantities are available to corporations, professional associations, and other organizations. For details and discount information, contact our special sales department.

Library of Congress Cataloging-in-Publication Data

Tremper, Terri, 1965–
    4 hands are better than 2 : a guide to original tandem massage / by Terri
Tremper and Tammi Tremper.
        p. ; cm.
    Includes bibliographical references and index.
    Summary: "A complete illustrated guide to tandem massage, 4 Hands Are Better Than 2 integrates contemporary therapeutic massage techniques (Ayurvedic mirror, deep tissue, Swedish, Shiatsu, and Reiki) into the ancient practice of tandem mirror massage"—Provided by publisher.
    ISBN 1-55643-611-4
    1. Massage therapy—Handbooks, manuals, etc.
[DNLM: 1. Massage—methods—Handbooks. WB 39 T791z 2006] I. Title: Four hands are better than two. II. Tremper, Tammi, 1965– III. Title.
RM721.T73 2006
615.8'22—dc22   2005034388

    1 2 3 4 5 6 7 8 9 DATA 12 11 10 09 08 07 06

To our Fam Club,
whose light guides us,
and
to our loyal clients of Polson, Montana,
whose light inspires us.

Our deepest fear is not that we are inadequate.
Our deepest fear is that we are powerful beyond measure.
It is our light, not our darkness, that most frightens us.
We ask ourselves, who am I to be brilliant, gorgeous, talented,
fabulous? Actually, who are you not to be?
You are a child of God. Your playing small does not serve the world.
There is nothing enlightened about shrinking so that other
people won't feel insecure around you.
We are all meant to shine, as children do. We were born to
make manifest the glory of God that is within us.
It is not just in some of us; it is in everyone.
And as we let our own light shine, we unconsciously
give other people permission to do the same.
As we are liberated from our own fear, our presence
automatically liberates others.

—MARIANNE WILLIAMSON,
A Return to Love: Reflections on the Principles of a
Course in Miracles, 1992 (also included within
Nelson Mandela's 1994 inaugural speech)

Acknowledgments

We are so blessed. We have had the honor and privilege of being influenced by so many incredible people in our personal lives and careers, both prior to and in massage therapy. We wish to extend our appreciation to the following people, without whom this book would have remained just an elusive idea:

At North Atlantic Books, Richard Grossinger, Susan Bumps, Emily Boyd, Melissa Mower, Suzanne Albertson, and the whole staff. To you, we are eternally grateful. You believed in the project immediately and supported us every step of the way.

To the Northwest School of Massage: director Jack Weaver, and teachers Amon Greene, Cathy Patillo, Marcus O'Crotty, and Renee Escobar, we thank you for the solid education and background you provided us in so many different modalities. You inspired our passion for massage and supplied us with all the tools necessary to succeed and shine. For more information about the school, see the reference listing at the back of the book.

To Fumiko Medford, who enthusiastically created the anatomical drawings for this book. We are fortunate to have such a talented friend.

To Frank Tremper for his outstanding photography. We are so thankful for your skills, patience, and kindness.

To Jake Szczukowski and Russell Williams, thank you for your joyful willingness to model for the numerous pictures in this book. Your enthusiasm and full cooperation made this undertaking fun and memorable.

To Debbie, Robyn, and Mom, thank you for your help, patience, and brilliant ideas during the photo shoots. Special thanks to Debbie Williams who also took some beautiful pictures.

To Carlisa London, our client and friend, who along with her husband, Paul, willingly suggested and allowed us to take pictures at their beautiful KOA campground in Polson (see reference list at the back of the book). We are so lucky to know you.

To Mary Anne Moseley, our cousin, thank you for giving us your immediate permission to use your gorgeous deck on the lake. You mean so much to us.

To Marie Noble, owner of The Style Depot, thank you for your unfailing encouragement and countless referrals. We treasure your friendship. To Marcie Motichka, hair stylist and friend, thanks for increasing the joy in the shop and keeping our hair looking good.

Our family and friends, the "Fam Club," who give our spirits unconditional love and steady encouragement. Words cannot express our love and gratitude. To our dad, whose earthly presence we miss, but who is so much of who we are and hope to be. To our mom, whose constant love and humor warms our hearts. To our brother, Frank, whose ingenuity and talent constantly amaze us. To Linda, who remains steadfast and always supportive. To our brother, Tim, whose gentle nature and humor remind us of Dad. To his wife, Kathy, and their three children, Timmy, Trisha, and Tessah, who bring joy beyond all measure. To our sister, Debbie, whose laughter and love ring in our hearts. To her husband, Bill, and their three children, Ryan married to Annie, Russell, and Robyn married to Jake, who constantly remind us that life is good. To our brother Tom, who freely gives from his heart and creates fun wherever he goes. To Mark, who adds joy to the family. To our Aunt Donna (Mom's twin) and Uncle Claude, who are the epitome of love and generosity, not to mention proliferation. To all the Huguet clan, with whom we share so many treasured moments. You bless us more than words could say. To all our relatives, thank you for your love and unending support. To all our dear friends, we love you.

Most of all, thank you to our clients in Polson, Montana. You bless us with your trust and share your spirit with us. You are our teachers.

Contents

B. Sample Fifteen-Minute Seated Tandem Massage Routine 153
(Combination of shiatsu, trigger point, and Swedish)

Introduction

Therapeutic massage is one of the fastest growing industries in the nation. During the past decade, people of all ages and lifestyles are flocking to alternative medicine to treat their physical, emotional, and spiritual pain. Massage is the leading spa treatment and the second leading alternative medicine modality in the United States today. Four-hands massage is the latest and the greatest for elite spa guests. Two therapists massaging one client at the same time—what could be more heavenly? This approach can be applied to therapeutic massage as well.

With an estimated 150,000 massage therapists in the United States, the importance of differentiating your practice from the competition is essential. Not only is tandem massage a specialty to pique client interest and referrals, it is also a way for clients to receive twice as much work in one hour as with standard one-therapist massage. In this fast-paced, high-stress society, clients need massage more than ever, yet many have difficulty finding the time for routine massage. When people overcome the time hurdle, they can effectively double the effects with tandem massage in the same amount of time. Tandem massage can also minimize the potential risks involved with practicing solo.

Massage has blossomed into hundreds of different modalities. Some types of massage focus on specific muscle groups, while others correct imbalances of energy and/or elements. Creative tandem massage can incorporate any or all of these massage modalities. Therapists will appreciate the increased profits, safety, and camaraderie that come with practicing in tandem, while clients will value the augmented healing. Reading this book will help you gain confidence in utilizing two therapists to achieve one treatment goal, while stimulating creativity to honor the vast and diverse kinds of massage practiced today.

The first half of *4 Hands Are Better Than 2* reveals fourteen steps to create successful tandem massage routines that utilize each therapist's unique talents, while addressing each client's distinct needs. In addition, the steps show therapists how to build a thriving business with increased and reliable profits, a steady stream of loyal clients, effective treatment of pain and dysfunction, and rewarding work that balances the mind, body, and spirit.

Part II offers a sample step-by-step integrative (Ayurvedic Mirror, deep tissue, Swedish, shiatsu, and Reiki), one-hour tandem routine, a sample ten- to fifteen-minute seated tandem routine, and a sample tandem subroutine for piriformis syndrome. Piriformis syndrome is a common condition caused by tightness of the lateral hip rotator muscles, namely the piriformis. Pain, numbness, or spasm results from impingement of the sciatic nerve, which is called "sciatica." Piriformis syndrome, misaligned vertebrae, or disc problems can cause sciatica.

Each step of the tandem routines and subroutine contains solid therapeutic techniques to target specific muscle groups. Each step is described in detail and photographed for easy application. The routines are comprised of synchronous and asynchronous components. The asynchronous components enable each therapist to address specific and variable client needs, while the synchronous components maintain the cohesiveness to keep every client balanced and fully relaxed.

PART I

Steps to Success with
Four-Hands Massage

Understand the Benefits of and Misconceptions about Tandem Massage

Discover the power and endless possibilities of tandem massage.

- Create a unique niche in the market that offers clients more than traditional massage.
- Develop a working relationship with another bodyworker that stimulates creativity and makes work twice the fun with nearly double the profits.
- The advantages of tandem massage versus standard massage are countless. Eight of the most distinct benefits will be explored and must be appreciated before you will be inspired to add this modality to your repertoire.
- Four common misconceptions will also be discussed in order to recognize client hesitancies to receive tandem bodywork.
- Because word-of-mouth is the most powerful marketing tool for massage therapy, quotes from our Tandem Touch Therapeutic Massage clients in Polson, Montana, are included to highlight the numerous benefits of tandem massage.
- Understanding these primary benefits and misconceptions is crucial in order to enhance your ability to "sell" your clientele on tandem massage and to increase your desire to redefine your current practice to include four-hands massage.

Double Your Healing Efficiency

With two therapists working in tandem, each client receives twice as much work in one session. The choreography of tandem massage scatters the client's attention. The client will be unable to focus both sets of movements, so she will "give in" more easily to a deep state of relaxation. Client J.F. notices, "With the tandem massage, it is easier to relax during the deep tissue parts because the other part feels so great that you can just let it happen."

If the client is able to concentrate on one set of movements, she will naturally choose the set that feels the best, which also enhances relaxation. Client A.V. confirms, "You two have such alike pressure and movements that it is hard to tell who is doing what . . . like a dance and you lose yourself in it." This increased state of relaxation augments the effectiveness of each massage stroke. With this amplified relaxation and twice the amount of bodywork, the therapeutic result is more than doubled.

Clients will notice an immediate, gratifying, and restorative outcome, which will increase the probability of regularly scheduled visits. The numerous benefits of bodywork are doubled with four-hands massage.

Effectively Double Your Time

Since each therapist has a full hour for just one half of the body, therapists no longer need to watch the clock in order to perform a full-body massage. Clients recognize the thoroughness of a massage performed by two trained therapists, rather than one. Massage therapist and client J.F. confirms, "I never leave feeling like 'I wish they would've done this or that.' . . . I feel like every muscle that needed attention got it." The need to prioritize work on numerous tight muscles is virtually eliminated because twice the time is created for each body part.

This "extra" time allows therapists to concentrate on specific conditions, while maintaining the ability to fit the traditional full-body massage into one session. Therapists can wait for each release without feeling rushed. The massage will naturally become more intuitive when time is not a prime motivator. In addition, therapists can use time more creatively, either in synchrony or as individual therapists within the tandem modality. Both client and therapist will profit from the more relaxed pace of tandem massage.

Balance Your Clients

Tandem massage strokes performed synchronously on each side of the body activate and balance the left and right hemispheres of the brain.

Craniosacral therapist and client S.O. remarks, "I don't know how you two do it, but I always feel so balanced and grounded after your massage." Ayurvedic practitioners have used Tandem Mirrored Massage for thousands of years to achieve balance of the three "doshas" or biological principles of the body (Chabot 2002, p. 8).

Client T.M. exclaims, "Wow! It is like a dance. I feel lighter than air!" The synchronized downward, or "apana vayu," strokes bring negative energy out of the body and promote tranquility and centering (Chabot 2002, p. 38). Client L.L. affirms, "To have two equally strong people work on you is an exquisite experience. . . . I always leave their massage room feeling more centered and at peace." When you incorporate these synchronous strokes into your tandem routine, your clients will feel better, lighter, grounded, centered, relaxed, and balanced.

Distinguish Your Business

Four-hands massage is a unique way to distinguish your practice from the competition. The need to be outstanding in the field is necessary for a thriving business. Often, experience and talent are not enough. Tandem massage differentiates your practice from your competitors. Potential clients have asked, "Four-hands massage? What could be better?" and "Two therapists at one time? Sign me up!" After her first tandem session, client K.S. mentioned, "On a scale of one to ten, your solo massages would be a ten, but your tandem massages would rate a fifty!"

These comments are powerful marketing tools for word-of-mouth referrals. Curiosity will stimulate more appointments and the tandem massage itself will turn one-timers into loyal clients. Client P.W. validates, "Each time my session is complete, I can't wait to come back again."

Decrease Your Personal Risk

With two therapists working together, susceptibility and vulnerability to crime against practitioners is drastically reduced, regardless of the genders involved. It creates a built-in buddy system for bodyworkers.

Four-hands massage is the answer to the potential dangers of practicing solo. Therapists breathe easier when scheduling an unknown client and appreciate the sense of safety that comes with working in tandem.

Double Nurturance

Another advantage of tandem massage is that the client will feel deeply nurtured. With two trained professionals working simultaneously to alleviate his pain, the client will feel cared for in a profound manner. Client L.L. substantiates, "Tammi and Terri are beautiful caregivers of my spirit." Physical, emotional, and spiritual pain is recorded in our bodies in hypertense muscles, chaotic or stagnant energy, structural alignment, and posture.

Every body needs to be nurtured in order to work through this pain on a conscious or subconscious level. Client J.B. corroborates, "They have a very positive energy and spirit that is very nurturing to the client." Massage communicates a gentle knowing and concern for each client's pain. Tandem massage doubles this message of nurturance.

Heighten Your Sense of Spirituality

Three is a venerated number in numerous religions and cultures. In Ayurveda, there are three "doshas" in the body, the Vata, Pitta, and Kapha. Countless traditions honor the Trinity of the Father, Son, and Holy Spirit. Contemporary spirituality and psychology acknowledges the power of the mind, body, and spirit. Client D.R. comments, "Your massage felt so spiritual." Client N.H. concurs, "That was heavenly." Two therapists working with one client equals three people in the treatment room. Tandem massage unites three people in the sacred process of healing.

Instant Second Opinion

Clients will profit from the wisdom of two trained therapists united in one treatment goal. When two therapists work in tandem, both therapists see, listen, and feel the needs of the client. When two practitioners brainstorm together, new techniques can be created to achieve a healing response that does not come from traditional approaches. Tandem massage stimulates creativity, which is the secret to a fulfilling career. Massage therapists can bounce ideas off one another to develop new techniques. Four-hands massage clients benefit from the knowledge and skills of two therapists in each session.

The "Too Confusing" Misconception

The most common client hesitancy in receiving tandem massage is the thought that four hands will be too confusing. Although completely understandable, the fact is that it is virtually impossible for the brain to focus on more than one place at a time. The movements of both therapists are noticed and appreciated by the body, but the brain can only acknowledge one or the other.

Rather than confusion, the response is one of letting go. Thoughts will transcend the bodywork of both therapists and drift to a meditative and relaxed state. As client L.L. explains, "At first, I was very apprehensive about having two people massage me at the same time. Once the massage began, I became lost in the rhythm and the motion of the massage." The idea of four-hands massage can seem overwhelming until it is actually experienced. Isn't that true with any new experience? Encourage your clients to take the chance on a new form of bodywork that may take them to a new level of relaxation, peacefulness, centeredness, and decreased muscular pain.

The "No Draping" Misconception

The second most common misconception about tandem massage is that little or no draping is used. With tandem massage, two body parts are uncovered at one time. However, this does not mean that the rest of the body is left uncovered. The greatest exposure during a tandem session occurs when the back and one leg are uncovered with the client in a prone position. The other leg and buttocks are covered. Give every client the option of wearing underwear or shorts to ensure client comfort, particularly for the first session. This misconception about draping techniques will be resolved when the client has actually experienced his first tandem massage.

The "Tantric" Misconception

Another misconception, although thankfully rare, is that "tandem" means "tantric," which implies a sensual component. Adding the words "therapeutic," "professional," and/or "treatment" to the business name or service easily remedies this mistaken belief. Document professional certifications and affiliations on your business cards and brochures.

Include several sentences about sexual misconduct on your intake form. Examples of intake forms with explanations of misconduct are included in professional massage association information packets available from Associated Bodywork and Massage Professionals and the American Massage Therapy Association. Hang educational certificates in the waiting area.

When a client calls to schedule an appointment, clarify that tandem means two trained professionals performing therapeutic massage techniques. If for any reason you feel that the potential client's interests are suspect, ask what type of massage he is interested in. If his response includes a specific desire for inner thigh, groin, and/or buttock massage, simply state that the purpose of your tandem massage is therapeutic and does not include a sexual or sensual component.

Regardless of his response, if your intuition signals any risk, do not book him an appointment. Most potential clients who believe that tandem is a sensual massage will understand as soon as the words "therapeutic" or "professional" are used. Fortunately, this misconception is very uncommon and usually remedied prior to scheduling.

The "Indulgent" Misconception

A fourth misconception is that tandem massage is an indulgent, purely relaxing spa treatment. Although tandem massage is most readily available in fancy spas, the therapeutic benefits far exceed simple relaxation.

Tandem massage balances the left and right hemispheres of the brain, enhances circulation and wellness, and treats muscular disorders and/or energy imbalances. Client C.L. verifies, "My back and neck always require a lot of attention and this was the first massage where those areas were done well, along with the rest of my body."

Tandem massage is a therapeutic treatment based on ancient Ayurvedic and contemporary therapeutic massage techniques. Client P.W. confirms, "The bodywork . . . has helped me immensely with my stress and headaches." The benefits of tandem massage far exceed "indulgence."

 STEP TWO

Imagine Yourself Working in Tandem

Imagine the possibilities and realities of how tandem massage can enliven your current massage practice. Try to glimpse into the everyday working situation of working in tandem. Think about the personal, professional, and financial ways that tandem massage would support you on a day-to-day basis.

Weigh the Tandem Option

Tandem massage will bring benefits to you, your clients, and your current practice. Reflect on the following questions:

- Are you prepared to work closely with another massage therapist?
- Would you enjoy learning new techniques and sharing your techniques with another bodyworker?
- Will you be agreeable to scheduling and coordinating time with another therapist?
- How do you feel about the possibility of sharing space and expenses?
- Are you ready to introduce yourself and your clients to a completely new experience?

- Do you want to increase your practice two-fold, establish a fiercely loyal client base, and create higher income?

Imagine All Business Responsibilities . . . Halved!

An especially nice benefit is that there are two people to divide business duties. One of you may enjoy returning phone calls, while the other could be better at charting. Expenses, insurance billing, scheduling clients, charting, organizing tax records, and other tasks can be shared. You and your associate can bounce ideas off one another to create methods that are more efficient.

Be open to learning where each other's strengths and interests are when it comes to managing the other business-related activities, so the tasks will be easier to assign and be more fun to accomplish. It's a win-win business situation. Quite possibly, you will still be doing an occasional one-therapist massage, during which your co-worker can input data in the computer or schedule clients, should you decide to become business partners.

Envision On-Site Tandem Massages

Four hands make lighter work. You carry only half of the equipment. No more second trips out to the car will be needed or the taking a risk of breaking your back while attempting to lug all your equipment in one trip. Two minds are more likely to find effective treatments for perplexing client symptoms than one occasionally feeble mind alone. Have coffee on your way back to the office. You saved time and have a colleague for conversation. You can be sure it will likely be twice as much fun and far more enlightening than your usual internal banter.

Visualize the Actual Massage

You and your partner will exude a calming confidence because you have a harmonious routine that allows ample time for every body part. You can actually work on every muscle that needs attention without feeling rushed. The pace is slow and relaxing to both of you and to your client.

Your client will feel satisfied knowing that all the areas that needed work got it. You and your co-worker conclude the session with a simultaneous foot and head massage that puts your client into a blissful state of glorious relaxation.

Your client is hooked and will rebook, asking, "How can I ever go back to having a normal massage?" You will smile and think, "How can I ever go back to being a solo therapist?" Four-hands massage is full of rewards, creative movements and moments, and pure enjoyment.

STEP THREE
Know Yourself and Your Fellow Bodyworker

This step will assist you in finding the right person with whom to combine your talents for tandem massage. Self-awareness and communication in this step will pave the way to a collaborative and symbiotic relationship to succeed in tandem massage.

Find the Right "Fit"

Trade massage with a potential associate for tandem massage. Let her experience your gifts. Recognize her gifts. Talk about the massages. Express your interest in doing four-hands massage and ask her to read the first two steps of this book. Discuss each other's thoughts. You will be working closely together, so it is important to enjoy each other's company and feel a mutual respect for one another's work. You do not necessarily need to practice the same type of massage, just types that would blend effectively.

Communication Is Key

You need to verbalize your preferences for the environment you like to create with your clients and the types of massage skills you wish to coordinate with your new associate. Discuss these insights with your perspective cohort and inquire about her skills, strengths, weaknesses, and preferences.

Try being direct when discussing things that annoy you and speak up about the things in massage that you are passionate about. Now is the time to discover and delve into each other's dreams and desires for your massage careers. Talk about all the business aspects. Your discussion will prompt a flow of excitement and energy with all the possibilities that await you when you begin practicing in tandem. Create a motto for your tandem work together to remind each other of your professional goals. For example, ours is "Two gentle spirits, four healing hands."

STEP FOUR
Develop Routines Based on Talents and Preferences

Recognize Your Gifts

To succeed, you must be able to celebrate and utilize each other's strengths and preferences. Bishop Desmond Tutu, 1984 Nobel Peace Prize winner, was recognized for his peaceful efforts to end the apartheid in South Africa. The African ubuntu theory recognizes each individual as crucial to the community because God gives every human being unique gifts. Tutu perceives these gifts as distinct from other individual's gifts, rather than one being superior to another (Battle 1997, p. 44–45). This negates the need for competition, while increasing our interdependence on one another. Thus, each gift is utilized for the fullest enrichment and greatest benefit of the community.

Utilize Your Unique Talents

In other words, help your associate to recognize and value her unique gifts and talents. She will do the same for you. You will both be empowered. Celebrate each other's gifts by creating routines that utilize your special talents. No competition exists between two therapists when each therapist is recognized by the other to possess unique talents. In this way, you will not rival each other. Instead, you will become aware of the ways in which you and your associate complement each other.

Be inspired to combine your talents in innovative ways to stimulate healing in your clients. Personal preferences must also be considered when generating your tandem routines for mutual contentment. Open communication is the key to developing creative and intuitive routines. Talents and preferences also lead to combinations of techniques to form shorter and/or more specialized sessions. For example, a thirty-minute reflexology treatment could be integrated with Swedish neck massage or a one-hour Reiki session with twice the healing energy. Your clients will benefit as you and your associate feel growing gratification from your work because your natural healing gifts are being explored and nurtured.

 STEP FIVE

Use Both Synchronous and Asynchronous Strokes

This step is the heart and art of our innovative approach to tandem massage. The advantages and disadvantages of routines comprised solely of either synchronous strokes or asynchronous strokes will be discussed. Let your tandem routines evolve and grow with a balance of both synchronous and asynchronous strokes—yin and yang, so to speak. The synchronous sequences provide a balancing rhythm, while the asynchronous sections allow each therapist time for solo work to meet specific client needs.

No Synchronous Strokes

Four-hands routines that have no mirrored movements generate a sense of disorganization and unease. This apprehension will be subtly expressed as an inability to fully relax, which will reduce the effectiveness of each massage stroke. Twice the work of a one-therapist massage will be achieved, but the therapeutic value will be less than if one therapist worked twice as long. Any two therapists with no prior experience in tandem massage could improvise their way through this type of session. However, the advantages of increased relaxation, balancing and grounding, and maximized stretches will not be achieved. Thus the potential therapeutic effectiveness of two therapists working in tandem will not be fully realized. When you add synchronous components to a routine of asynchronous strokes, your client will experience the full reward of two therapists working in tandem.

Completely Synchronous Routines

Synchronous tandem massage has the distinct advantage of balancing the left and right hemispheres of the brain, which induces a remarkable sense of relaxation and grounding. The client will enjoy the massage and be impressed by the ability of the two therapists to remain in sync, but may feel as though his specific needs are secondary to the routine and are not adequately addressed. This type of tandem massage then becomes a "special" treatment, but not a regularly scheduled treatment necessary for pain management.

True Ayurvedic Mirror Massage is a beautiful art form that is not completely synchronous and carefully addresses client need with Ayurvedic principles and medicine. For more information on Ayurvedic Mirror Massage, go to www.sacredstonehealing.com. Unfortunately, most spa tandem massages borrow the synchronous strokes, but do not address individual needs with the ancient, healing medicine of Ayurveda.

The key to repeat and loyal clientele is the ability to meet each client's changing needs. Completely synchronous routines cannot readily adapt to these variables. One recipient of a completely synchronized tandem massage described the massage as invigorating, "like going through a carwash." The therapists were unable to vary their routine to fit the client's specific needs, so the client felt as though the massage was mechanical. Every body is treated with the same routine. This is suitable for clients who want to experience a four-hands massage, but not appropriate for repeat clientele and/or injury treatment massage. By adding asynchronous components to a synchronous routine, the benefit of balancing is maintained and the ability to meet client need is gained.

Combination of Synchronous and Asynchronous Strokes

By blending both synchronous and asynchronous movements, the routine will be cohesive and balancing with the distinct advantage of effortless flexibility to meet clients' individual and changing needs. The flexibility lies in the blocks of time dedicated to asynchronous strokes. When the two therapists are not performing mirrored strokes, specific muscle group work can be done. By including synchronous, mirrored strokes in the routine, many of the benefits of Ayurvedic tandem massage are maintained.

In the sample routines, both therapists begin with synchronous strokes. An asynchronous block of time follows, which allows each therapist time for therapeutic techniques to meet specific client needs. Then both therapists perform a synchronous stroke before moving to the next section. The synchronous movement can be as simple as stroking downward from the shoulders to the fingertips. In Ayurvedic massage, this downward direction is called "apana vayu." Apana vayu strokes are used to move negative energy away from the center of the body down and out through the extremities (Chabot 2002, p. 38). This easy stroke will provide balancing and grounding, as well as a connecting and soothing stroke before moving on to another asynchronous section.

The use of both asynchronous and synchronous blocks of time allows each therapist time to work on specific muscles or energy constrictions, while providing a balanced and cohesive tandem massage. Creative tandem routines that blend both synchronous and asynchronous movements achieve the maximum client benefit, while enhancing therapist satisfaction.

STEP SIX

Be Mindful of Each Other's Movements

Each therapist must be aware of her associate's strokes in order to enhance her work rather than hinder it. Small considerations make a big difference, both in the effectiveness of the treatment and in the ongoing working relationship of the therapists. Tandem therapists need to be both intuitive and candid about all aspects, i.e., be aware of what works and what does not, in order to attain the benefits of a healthy working relationship.

Be Considerate

Even during the asynchronous components, each therapist must be considerate of her associate. You must avoid broad strokes that cause tissue movement in the location where your fellow bodyworker is doing deep tissue. For instance, when one therapist is doing linear friction on the multifidi of the lower back, the second therapist must avoid broad movements on the gluteus muscles because it could cause the first therapist to roll off the hypertense multifidi abruptly and prematurely.

Complement Each Other's Strokes

In addition, if you notice your partner is performing a passive stretch, you may be able to enhance that stretch with a complementary movement. For example, when the client is in a prone position and your associate is lifting the leg to stretch the ilio-psoas, you could enhance that stretch with a linear stroke up the longissimus. (Figure 6.1) Gentle, non-verbal communication with your associate during the massage will help in this process until an intuitive knowing is realized.

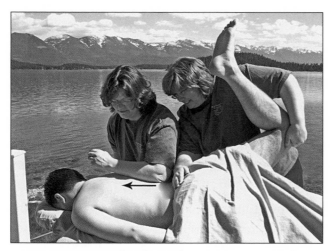

Figure 6.1. Passive stretch with complementary massage stroke

STEP SEVEN
Practice for Compatibility, Rhythm, and Client Comfort

Practice Sessions
Set up at least seven practice sessions at no charge with friends or loyal clients who will offer constructive criticism and positive feedback. It is crucial for therapists and clients to have ample opportunity to discuss specific movements at the exact time that the movements are performed. Even the most compatible and intuitive therapists with the best-planned routines have a learning curve.

Ask for Candid Feedback
Inform the practice clients that you and your associate are trying to polish a four-hands routine, so you will be asking for their feedback during and after the massage. Tell them that you and your associate will also be talking to one another during the massage in order to coordinate movements. Stress the importance of the client's immediate and candid comments about what feels good and what does not.

Voice Your Thoughts

After the first few massages, you and your fellow therapist will begin to notice a rhythm and be able to pinpoint which techniques work well when performed simultaneously and which do not. You will also notice movements that your associate does that detract from your work rather than enhance it. Mention these things right away, instead of waiting until the end of the massage. Keep in mind that your associate may enlighten you with considerations that you could make to improve the situation as well.

It is more time-consuming and ineffectual to explain, or even remember, than to simply blurt out feedback to your associate during the practice massages.

If this step is skipped, many avoidable irritations will continue with every massage because the therapists and clients had no opportunity in the moment to talk about exactly what bothers them. Silent annoyance is not conducive to creative growth and client healing. Relying on discussion afterward is ineffectual at best. Waiting thwarts memory, so the annoyance will be forgotten until it happens again.

Modify Your Routine

View these sessions as the learning sessions that they are and be willing to accept criticism from both the client and your associate. Both therapists must be willing to voice concerns and make changes even though much time and consideration have already been invested in developing the routine. Straightforward and honest communication in the beginning stages of your tandem working relationship will create an accepting environment capable of growth and creativity throughout the course of your practice together.

STEP EIGHT
Let the Body Speak

Cycles of Seasons

In his book, *Let Your Life Speak,* Parker Palmer uses the cycles of the seasons as a metaphor of life (2002). Autumn is a season of transformation, winter brings solitude and quiet clarity, spring promises hope and new growth, and summer brings abundance and community. He reminds us of theologian Thomas Merton's words, "There is in all visible things ... a hidden wholeness" (1989, p. 506). Palmer explains, "In the visible world of nature, a great truth is concealed in plain sight: diminishment and beauty, darkness and light, death and life are not opposites. They are held together in the paradox of 'hidden wholeness.'" (2000, p. 99).

Recognize the Wholeness

As bodyworkers, we perceive these paradoxes as a creative tension between healthy tissue and distressed tissue, health and infirmity, strength and frailty, comfort and pain, life and death. We cannot deny the connection between the body, mind, and spirit in the balance of these conflicting states. It is in the recognition of these states that we find wholeness.

The celebration and acknowledgment of these dichotomies is at the heart of the bodyworker's practice. If clients deny their pain, they would never seek help to achieve a better state of health. If we do not recognize these opposite states within our clients and ourselves, our practices will stagnate. We will offer a massage that never adapts to changing physical and emotional needs. We will then be refusing to celebrate the seasons of growth, death, and rebirth.

Our bodies, our practices, our routines, our clients' bodies, our clients' needs, and all the relationships in between will cycle through seasons. As bodyworkers, we need to let the body speak of these seasons and respond with a gentle knowing that we can see the hidden wholeness.

This provides a sense of deep nurturing to our clients and to ourselves, which facilitates self-healing.

Listen to the Body

When you are comfortable working in tandem, you will suddenly begin to notice and be able to listen to the client's body again, as you did when you were working solo. The joy of a good routine with periods of asynchronous movements is the extra time you can take on a hypertense muscle, fibrous adhesion, or stuck energy that is not specifically included in the regular routine. The routine itself becomes the vehicle for extra time to let the body speak to us. Your work will be become more focused when you listen to each muscle and how it functions with the rest of the body. Appreciating the balance of the muscle groups and energy in relation to emotional and spiritual factors is essential to recognize the needs as well as the wholeness and unique rhythms of the body.

Focus Your Awareness

All massage therapists are susceptible to distractive thoughts during the tranquility of a massage. Focused work on the distinct needs of each muscle group and/or energy imbalances will automatically reduce your susceptibility to distraction. By bringing your awareness to the point at which your body or energy field meets the client's, you can allow yourself to feel connected to the client's body. Thoughtfully feel each subtle nuance beneath the skin or within the energy field.

Let your intuition guide you. Envision the muscle beneath your hands and imagine the effect and response you wish to create. With work that is focused, distractions are virtually eliminated because the old routine becomes new with each client's different muscle characteristics. Be diligent in checking that you are grounded. The body will speak to us if we allow ourselves to be fully present to each subtlety at every point of contact in each moment that we are entrusted and blessed with the client's permission to touch.

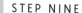

STEP NINE

Utilize Four Hands to Maximize Stretches

Stretches enhance the effects of massage by retraining contracted and shortened muscle groups. Two therapists working in tandem can maximize the lengthening response of the muscle. Certified Advanced Rolfer and author Art Riggs explains in his book, *Deep Tissue Massage: A Visual Guide to Techniques,* "... if a tight muscle is placed in an easy stretch near its end range, when the muscle relaxes, it will lengthen ... this educates the muscle stretch receptors to re-establish a new definition of what its resting length is" (2002, p. 17). Combining a stretch with simultaneous deep tissue or a gentle relaxation stroke will encourage muscle lengthening. (Figure 9.1)

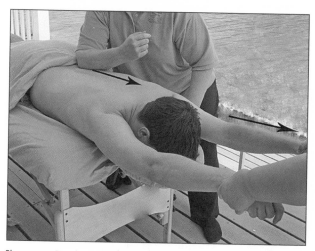

Figure 9.1. Passive stretch combined with deep tissue

Combining two stretches at the opposite ends of the muscle groups or on the same muscle bilaterally will also augment the lengthening response. (Figure 9.2)

Another effective way to lengthen a muscle is to anchor the muscle at one end, while performing a linear stroke in the opposite direction.

The first therapist can anchor the insertion site, while the second therapist uses both hands to perform the linear stroke away from the anchor. (Figure 9.3)

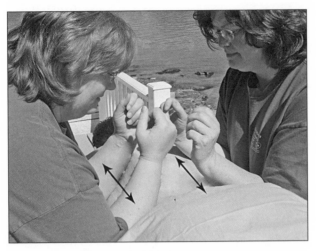

Figure 9.2. Combine two stretches

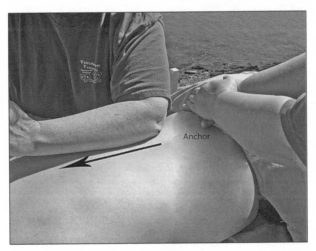

Figure 9.3. Muscle anchor with linear stroke in opposite direction

Work with each other to develop coordinated movements that have a synergic result. Spontaneous and creative movements will often occur when each therapist is aware of the movements and intention (e.g., muscle lengthening) of their fellow bodyworker. New combinations of movements will keep creativity flowing.

STEP TEN

Develop Subroutines for Common Conditions

By developing subroutines, treatment for common conditions will become second nature. Before the massage begins, you and your associate will know exactly how the massage will progress simply based on client assessment and/or history. This optimizes the efficiency of the session by removing the indecision during the massage of which therapist does what and when. The sample subroutine for piriformis syndrome, beginning on page 180, illustrates this concept. Your confidence will soar as you solidify your treatment options. In this way, your full-body tandem massages can effortlessly incorporate injury treatment in the traditional one-hour session.

STEP ELEVEN

Listen to Your Client

Listening to your client's verbal and nonverbal communication is crucial for repeat and loyal clientele. With two caring and listening therapists, clients will feel doubly nurtured. Tandem therapists must guard against any communication with one another that draws their attention away from the client. All verbal communication should include your client.

Respond to Feedback

Clients will have specific preference or indifferences specific to the tandem routine. Encourage feedback by acknowledging that each client has unique thoughts about what feels good and what does not. Nonverbal communication is often the method bodyworkers must rely on to receive information about preferences and dislikes. A giggle may indicate that the client is uncomfortable. A sigh or groan usually indicates a pleasurable sensation or getting on the spot that is problematic. Listen carefully for any verbal or nonverbal signs of uneasiness in order to maximize client comfort and security by modifying the routine.

Actively Listen

Listen with your ears and your heart to whatever the client talks about while she is on and off the table. Your client will notice if you're only half listening. This is your client's time. Offer her your undivided attentive care, not only to her body, but to her mind as well. Words can convey an emotional meaning to the body's tension patterns.

Help your client become more aware of her body and of the fact that emotions, thought patterns, stress, and trauma affect the body. Respond with gentleness in your voice and touch. By thoughtfully listening to your client's words and bodies, you communicate to her that she is an important human being who is worthy of attention and care. In doing so, you will not only help the client to heal herself, but your compassion and fulfillment will grow.

Nurture Client During an Emotional Release

The mind, body, and soul connection is a powerful force. Massage often brings emotions to the surface to be let go. If your client begins to cry, respond with soft words of acceptance. Let him know that crying is a normal response to bodywork. Acknowledge his tears by sitting at the head of the table. Gently place your hands on his face and wipe away the tears with your thumbs. Your associate could embrace your client's heart by placing one hand softly on his chest and sliding her other hand beneath his upper back. (Figure 11.1) Alternatively, your associate could sit at foot of table and hold client's ankles. This facilitates the flow of healing energy from head to toe. (Figure 11.2) Allow your client to feel your compassion and give him ample time to work through the emotions that can accompany bodywork.

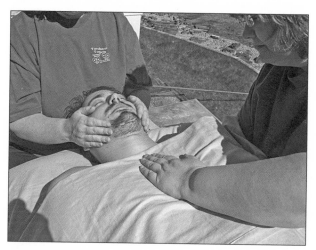

Figure 11.1. Nurture an emotional release

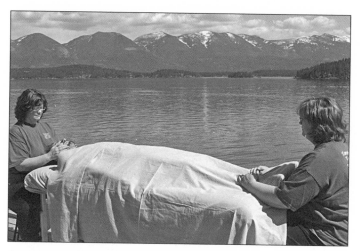

Figure 11.2. Healing energy from head to toe

Develop a Refocusing Phrase

Even the most attentive and focused therapists are subject to an occasional distractive thought. A refocusing phrase may be helpful to bring your attention back to your work and client. Ideally, the phrase should facilitate centering and grounding, while stating your intention in a few thoughtful words or sounds.

Reiki therapists often use "Se Ki Re," while Ayurvedic practitioners often say, "Hari Aum" or "aaahhh" (Chabot 2002, p. 11). These phrases work for them because they understand the powerful meaning behind the sounds. Massage therapists must develop a personal refocusing phrase that will work for them. For example, Tammi silently says, "Please bring healing and balancing energy, thank you." Terri states to herself, "God's healing love." A refocusing phrase will enable you to reconnect and be ready to listen and respond to the balance of the mind, body, and spirit.

STEP TWELVE
Market Your Tandem Massage

The following marketing strategies will stimulate immediate referrals at minimal cost. The easy-to-implement tips are designed to establish professional relationships, while boosting referrals and profits.

Discuss the Benefits of Tandem Massage

Word-of-mouth is an extremely powerful marketing tool. Use it to your advantage. Inform your clients and friends of the tremendous benefits of tandem massage. Create your own brochure or flyer that introduces each therapist and describes the benefits of tandem massage. Convey the special talents that each bodyworker brings to the table, as well as background and education.

Adjust Prices to Be Competitive *and* Profitable

You may wish to offer a client's first tandem session at a discounted rate or even a one-time price equal to that of your current solo therapist rate. This will introduce your clients to tandem massage and hopefully get them "hooked." If you do choose to offer a discount, you must be very clear about the regular price and that this is a first-time, one-time only price. Your clients will not fully appreciate the offer unless you are clear about the regular price. You do not want to fall into the trap of an "introductory" price that is then difficult to adjust.

In metropolitan areas, the price for tandem massage can be twice as much as a standard, one-therapist massage. The time saved in getting twice as much work done in one hour is worth the extra money. In more rural and/or low-income areas, the tandem price needs to be more than the going rate for a standard massage, but not quite double. The price must be low enough to stimulate increased referrals for a specialized service, low enough to establish repeat clientele, and high enough to increase profitability.

You can adjust the price to fit your needs. The advantage of tandem massage in both rural and urban communities is creating a niche that distinguishes your practice from other massage therapists in the area.

Inspire Media Coverage by Writing a Press Release

Newspapers will often print an article about a business new to the area at no charge. This is an excellent way to obtain publicity at no cost. Even if your business is well-established, tandem massage is a new service and just may provide a different enough angle to attract media attention. Include your experience, credentials, business phone number, hours, the regular tandem massage price, and possibly a one-time introductory price for tandem massage.

Give Every Client a Bottle of Water

More than ever, people are aware of the health benefits of drinking water. Increased water consumption is crucial after a massage to flush out the toxins and reduce muscle soreness. By giving water to your clients, you are encouraging them to drink more water and telling them that you care about their health. Water is far less expensive than giving away pens or notepads. Print labels with your business name, location, and phone number on regular or colored paper and cut it to size with a paper cutter. Use glue sticks to adhere the label to the water bottle. Clients will carry the water out with them and often refill it. The bottle then becomes a topic of conversation, thus spreading word-of-mouth referrals.

One word of caution: Do not sell the water with your label over the original label. This could get you into trouble. Give the water bottles away to avoid any legal ramifications. If you would like to sell water bottles with your logo, you must contact the water company. Many of our clients take their water bottles with them wherever they go and become a healthy, walking, water-drinking advertisement for our tandem massage.

Deliver Water Bottles, Brochures, and Business Cards to Area Businesses

Walk around town and stop in to as many businesses as you can. It really does not matter what type of business it is. All bodies benefit from massage. Face-to-face meetings create lasting impressions. Questions can be answered immediately. You become a friendly face instead of just another name on a card. Massage is a personal service, so people need to feel a connection and sense of security with the therapists.

An informal, unplanned meeting goes a long way toward forming a lasting connection. Even if the people you meet do not become your clients, they will remember you when one of their friends mentions a sore back. Give your hair stylist, pet groomer, physician, chiropractor, dentist, and any other people you do business with ten or so of your business cards to pass out for you. Do the same for them. Keep them stocked with your cards and show your appreciation when they refer someone by adding the name of the person they referred to their reward card. When either ten of their referrals come for a massage, or they receive ten massages, they will get a free massage as a bonus.

Send Out On-Site Seated Tandem Massage Information

On-site seated massage for local businesses is a wonderful service. Employers who allow a fifteen-minute break to include chair massage will notice decreased stress, reduction in repetitive motion injuries, and increased productivity in their employees. The employer can pay for this health benefit for each employee, the employees can pay individually, or create a combination of the two. The employer will already have the necessary information to make an informed decision. Stress the health benefits of regular on-site seated massage. Ask if you could meet with him or schedule an on-site seated massage session.

Thank Those Who Made Referrals

When a new client comes in for a tandem massage, be sure to ask who referred him to you. Include this question on your client intake form. As soon as you can, pick up the phone and call the person who referred your new client. Tell the referring people that you have a reward program and that you have started a card for them. After ten referrals and/or massages, they will get a free tandem massage. Expressing your gratitude is a wonderful opportunity to stimulate a warm conversation and has the extra bonus of encouraging more referrals. If the referring person has not had a tandem massage, this phone call acts as an invitation.

 STEP THIRTEEN

Take Care of Your Fellow Bodyworker

Self-care is necessary for long, prosperous careers in bodywork. Healthcare providers are notorious for taking care of others, while neglecting their own needs. When two therapists work together, taking care of your co-worker can accomplish the task of self-care.

Give Each Other a Weekly Massage

Massage exchanges should be scheduled every week with your fellow bodyworker. This time is beneficial for the health purposes of each therapist for the exchange of ideas and feedback on techniques.

Provide Daily Hand and Arm Care

In addition, therapists working together can work on each other's hands every day and develop short stretching, grounding, and clearing routines before stepping into the massage room. The following suggestions for daily hand and arm care take just a short time and will extend your pain-free bodywork careers. Most steps can easily be performed on yourself as well.

Daily Hand and Arm Care Steps:

1. Loosen wrist joint by holding it with both hands. Jostle gently and rotate in a bicycle fashion. (Figure 13.1)

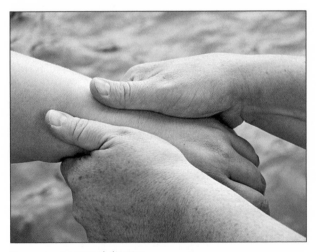

Figure 13.1. Wrist mobilization

2. In a snake-like fashion, extend and flex wrist while using your thumb and index fingers to realign joints. Exert pressure toward elbow with thumbs and toward hand with your index fingers. (Figure 13.2)

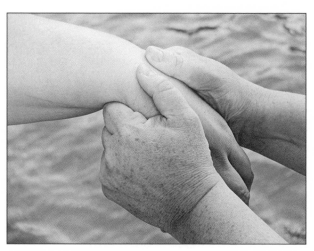

Figure 13.2. Re-align wrist joints

3. Invert partner's hand, so her palm is up. Place your little finger between her index and middle fingers. Place the little finger of your other hand between her ring and little fingers. Support your associate's hand with your other fingers. (Figure 13.3) Move your little fingers gently apart to stretch her hand.

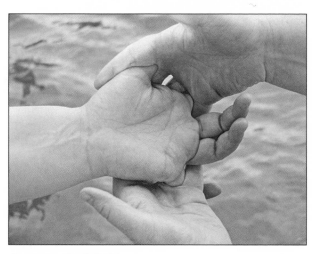

Figure 13.3. Hand stretch

4. Press in at the center of the heel of palm with both your thumbs. Glide to sides of hand to stretch palm muscles. Move toward fingers and repeat. Repeat to knuckles and back to heel of hand. (Figure 13.4)

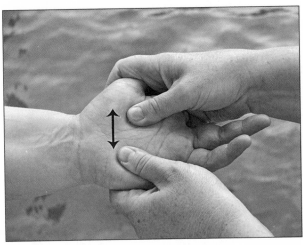

Figure 13.4. Gliding and stretching palm muscles

5. Support your associate's hand by placing one of your hands underneath her palm-up hand. Use your knuckle or thumb of your other hand to massage the thumb muscles thoroughly. Begin by placing your knuckle or pad of thumb between the first and second metacarpal bones close to the thumb and carpometacarpal joint. Follow the medial border of the first metacarpal and stroke out to the web of the thumb. The opponens pollicis muscle inserts at the lateral side of the thumb metacarpal and originates at the flexor retinaculum (the connective tissue across the front of the wrist). This muscle opposes the thumb. Use short strokes all around the base of the thumb. (Figure 13.5)

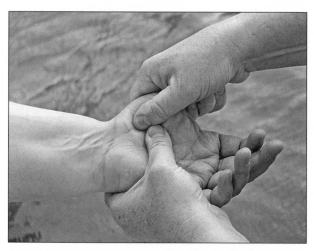

Figure 13.5. Massage opponens pollicis thumb muscle

6. Turn your associate's hand over (palm down). Place your
   thumb, knuckle, or fingertip between each knuckle (metacarpophalangeal joint). Apply pressure and stroke down toward
   wrist between each metacarpal to the carpal bones. (Figure
   13.6) Pay particular attention to the thumb metacarpal.

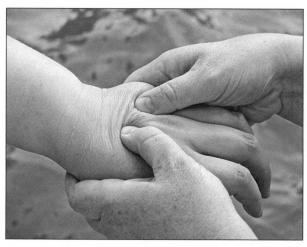

Figure 13.6. Linear strokes on dorsum of hand

7. Interlock your fingers with hers. Hold her forearm with your other hand. Pull your hands apart to create space in the wrist joint and stretch her fingers back. (Figure 13.7)

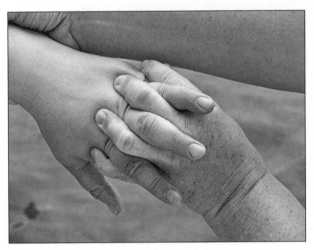

Figure 13.7. Finger/hand stretch

8. Pull each finger and thumb to create space in the joints. Grip with your index and middle fingers. (Figure 13.8)

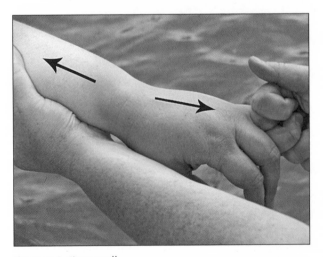

Figure 13.8. Finger pull

9. With your associate's palm down, use your knuckles to perform circular friction of wrist extensor muscles in forearm. (Figure 13.9) Begin with knuckles in center of associate's forearm just above wrist. Create small circles with knuckles while moving slowly up to elbow. Repeat on the ulnar and radial sides.

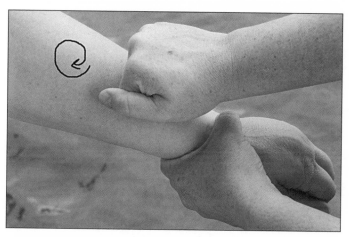

Figure 13.9. Circular friction of wrist extensors

10. Move back to wrist. Center thumbs just above wrist and slide thumbs away from each other for transverse friction of wrist extensors in forearm. Move up to elbow. (Figure 13.10)

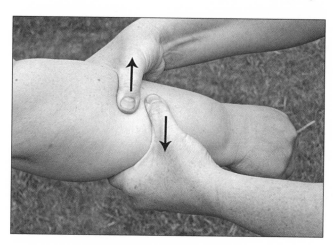

Figure 13.10. Transverse friction of wrist extensors

11. Use one or all knuckles for linear friction of wrist extensors in forearm. Place your knuckle just above your associate's wrist and slowly slide up the center of her forearm to her elbow. Flex her wrist to create a stretch to maximize the effect of the deep tissue strokes. Repeat on the ulnar and radial sides. (Figure 13.11)

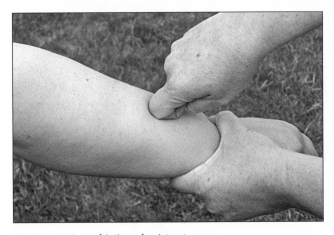

Figure 13.11. Linear friction of wrist extensors

12. With your associate's palm still down and wrist flexed, use your knuckles to perform deep tissue above and below elbow. This will affect many of the major muscle groups in the forearm and upper arm. Keep your knuckles straight as you use short strokes above and below the elbow. Pay particular attention to the origin of wrist extensors on the lateral epicondyle of humerus. (Figure 13.12)

13. Turn your associate's palm up. Extend wrist to add a stretch. Use short strokes with straight knuckles at the associate's anterior medial epicondyle of humerus (ulnar side of elbow). Repeat multiple times, moving slightly each time. This is the common origin of the major flexors of the wrist. (Figure 13.13) Move above and below the elbow to affect the major muscle attachments.

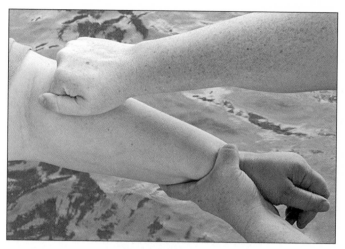

Figure 13.12. Deep tissue of extensor origin

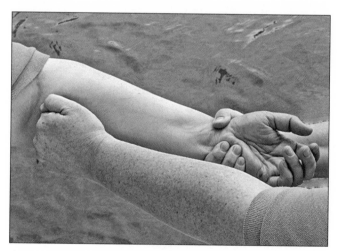

Figure 13.13. Deep tissue of flexor origin

14. Soothe entire arm with petrissage.

15. Repeat on your associate's other hand and arm.

16. Allow associate to stretch her extensors and flexors of both
    arms and thumbs before proceeding. (Figures 13.16a, 13.16b,
    and 13.16c) Be careful not to overstretch wrist. Hold each

stretch for thirty seconds. Hold palm of hand near knuckles, not near tips of fingers, to protect fingers and joints.

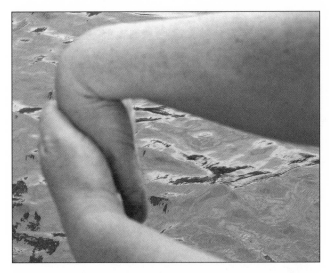

Figure 13.16a. Extensor stretch (palm down, push wrist down)

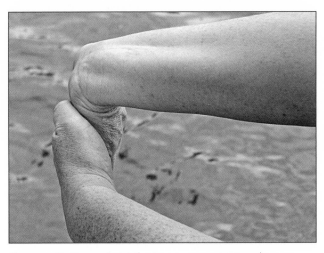

Figure 13.16b. Flexor stretch (palm up, pull wrist down)

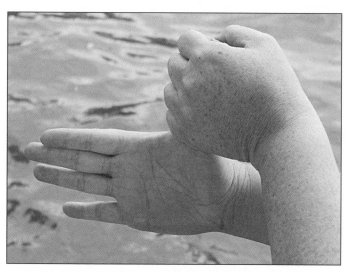

Figure 13.16c. Thumb stretch (keep wrist straight)

17. Switch roles and follow all steps, allowing your associate to
    work on your hands and arms.

In taking care of yourself and your partner, you will extend your
massage careers and maintain a professional and healthy working relationship.

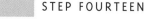 STEP FOURTEEN

Be Creative

Every massage is a living work of art. Each therapist has her own unique
way of expressing her individuality and purpose through her touch.
Every session should be viewed as a blessed opportunity to express yourself. The body is sacred. Communicate your reverence to each client.
Create flowing movements with a confident, soft touch. Move at a
peaceful, slow pace. Use comforting, gentle words. Give undivided,
focused attention and energy. Work with healing, loving intention. Give
your client a part of you. Let him experience your love of your art and
of humanity.

By using your talents creatively to fulfill the needs of your clients, you stimulate your own problem-solving skills and generate innovative work. This is crucial for a long and gratifying career in bodywork. Burnout in any career occurs when creativity and self-expression are suppressed. See each client as a unique opportunity to meet his specific needs using your whole toolbox of skills.

In tandem or solo massage, routines can become just that: routine, with little or no variation. They can become like mass reproductions of art instead of an original. By intermixing asynchronous blocks of time with synchronous blocks of time, creativity in tandem massage is easily achieved. In fact, the possibilities for the addition of new techniques are doubled. Two therapists can combine strokes and modalities to create powerful new treatments. Reflexology could be performed simultaneously with Reiki. Imagine the effectiveness of reflexology point stimulation coupled with healing energy to the corresponding organ!

Creativity need not be smothered by a tandem routine. On the contrary, let the routines that you create stimulate your ingenuity and originality. You will soon discover the endless possibility, power, and art of tandem massage.

PART II

Step-by-Step Sample Four-Hands Routines

O ur hope is that these routines will jumpstart your tandem massage skills, and also stimulate your creativity to produce your own custom routines. Please insert your own techniques into the asynchronous sections to make these sample routines your own. The routines do not represent the correct or only way to perform tandem massage, but they have worked for us. We trust that you will find them helpful as you begin to assimilate tandem massage into your practice. We highly recommend *Ayurvedic Mirror Massage* by Karyn Chabot and *Deep Tissue Massage: A Visual Guide to Techniques* by Art Riggs.

A. Sample One-Hour Integrative Massage
(Combination of Ayurvedic Mirror, Swedish, deep tissue, shiatsu, and Reiki)

This is our most requested massage. The synchronous and asynchronous components are designated at the beginning of each step. Please add and subtract deep tissue strokes in the asynchronous sections as needed for each particular client. Stretches are incorporated throughout the routine to enhance the effectiveness of the massage. The deep tissue massage strokes are balanced with soothing strokes that enable the client to remain completely relaxed.

Please Note: "Synchronous" means that the therapists perform identical movements on either side of the body at the same time. "Asynchronous" means that the movements of each therapist are not choreographed to match the other therapist, but are performed at same time. The two therapists are designated as "T1" and "T2." *Synchronous sections are written in italics,* while asynchronous sections are in plain text.

Steps 1–4. Back, Shoulders, Posterior Legs, and Buttocks

1. SYNCHRONOUS—T1 AND T2 PALM DOWN POSTERIOR BODY

T1—Begin on client's left side

T2—Begin on client's right side

T1 and T2—Position hands with palms down on either side of the spine between the scapulae. (Figure A-1.1)

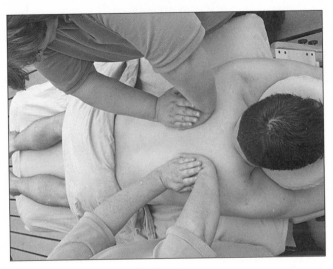

Figure A-1.1. *Hand position for first step*

Ask the client to take in a deep breath and let it out slowly. T1 and T2 press down with both hands gently at first, but firmly. Reposition hands farther down the spine and compress again. (Figure A-1.2) Time the compressions with the client's breathing, compress as the client exhales, and reposition hands during inhalation. Continue synchronous compressions down the posterior side of the body to the feet. Yang energy flows downward primarily along the posterior and outer surfaces. By moving from the upper back to the feet, the yang meridians are followed.

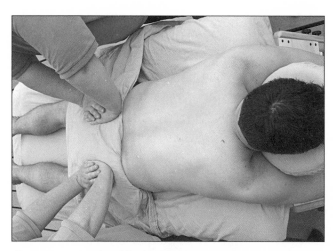

Figure A-1.2. *Four-hand back compressions*

2. SYNCHRONOUS—*T1 and T2 "BRUSH" DOWN SIDES OF BODY*

T1 and T2 place tips of fingers on either side of the top of the head and brush down both sides of the body simultaneously from head to toe to reset the parasympathetic nervous system and bring negative energy out through the feet. This movement is done with light pressure and relatively quick speed. (Figure A-2.1)

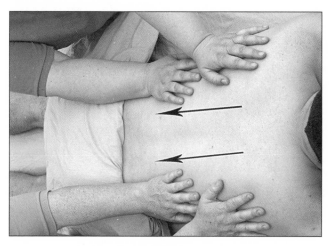

Figure A-2.1. *Brushing down sides of body*

3. ASYNCHRONOUS—T1 BACK AND SHOULDERS, T2 POSTERIOR LEGS
AND BUTTOCKS

T1—Uncover the back and tuck sheet gently under client's hip with palm facing downward. Begin back and shoulder work. (Figure A-3.1) T2—Uncover the right lower extremity. Pull sheet between legs and upward under hip. Begin work on right lower extremity and buttock. (Figure A-3.1)

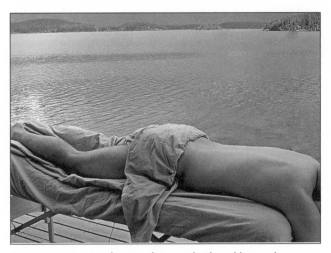

Figure A-3.1. Draping for asynchronous back and leg work

T1—**Back Work.** Begin with effleurage to spread the oil. Progress to petrissage. Then use inferior forearm to perform circular friction beginning at the iliac crest. (Figure A-3.2) Move in small circular movements to the axilla and back down.

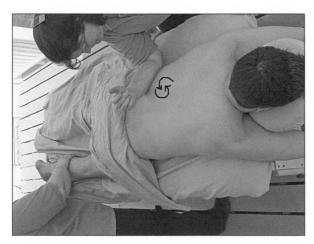

Figure A-3.2/ Circular friction on trunk

Next, apply cross-fiber friction to the latissimus dorsi and quadratus lumborum using a sawing motion with the forearm beginning at posterior superior iliac spine (PSIS) to axilla and back down. Using the same sawing motion, move forearm up to axilla again. "Windshield wiper" the axillary region by planting your elbow on the table and moving your forearm back and forth to relax the latissimus dorsi and teres major. (Figure A-3.3) Bring your forearm straight up and down. Slide down side of body to PSIS.

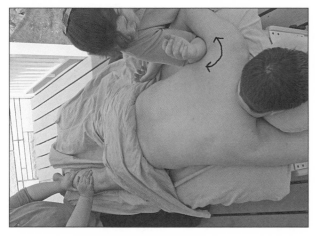

Figure A-3.3. "Windshield wiper" at axilla

At PSIS, saw up and down for cross-fiber friction on the origin of the quadratus lumborum. (Figure A-3.4) Next, use point of elbow for deeper penetration.

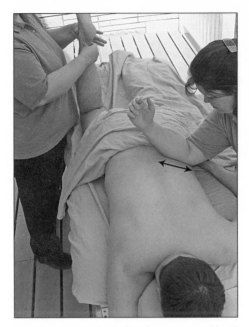

Figure A-3.4. Quadratus lumborum cross-fiber friction

Next, move elbow point from lumbar sacrum up along spine for linear friction of the erector spinae. (Figure A-3.5) This stroke coincides with T2 ilio-psoas stretch.

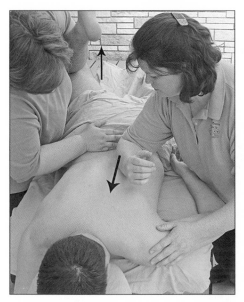

Figure A-3.5. Coordinated erector spinae linear friction and iliopsoas stretch

Let elbow roll off shoulder. Loosen tissue around scapula with petrissage. Take client's left arm and swing it freely on the side of the table. Then place the client's arm on the table with hand and wrist on or near the iliac crest. Position your superior hand under the client's left shoulder. Lift shoulder with left hand to passively flex the rhomboids, while slowly sinking right hand into tissue under the scapula. Maintain inward pressure while gliding up and down the medial border of the scapula to access and work the serratus posterior superior. (Figure A-3.6)

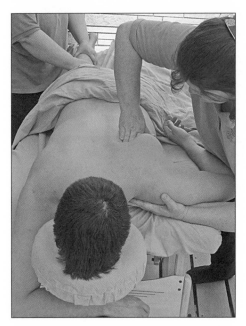

Figure A-3.6. Serratus posterior superior work

Repeat several times until tissue softens. Gently rock the shoulder back down to the table and then use both hands to compress the scapula. Maintain pressure while gliding out to the shoulder and down the arm to fingertips. Petrissage the entire arm beginning at the wrist and working up to the shoulder. (Figure A-3.7)

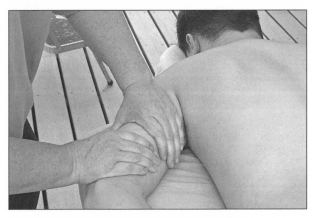

Figure A-3.7. Petrissage posterior upper extremity

Perform transverse friction by using wringing motion with hands from elbow to shoulder. (Figure A-3.8)

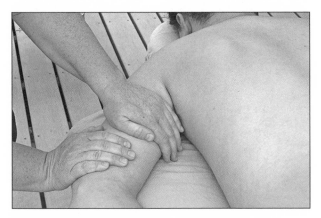

Figure A-3.8. Transverse friction on triceps

Sink thumbs or elbow point into tricep just above elbow and slowly move up the muscle to perform linear friction. (Figure A-3.9) If you use your thumbs, support them with loosely closed fists. Use as little pressure as necessary. This is generally tender. If no linear friction is needed on the tricep, simply start closer to the shoulder. Slowly glide up over posterior deltoid and through supraspinatus along superior border of scapula. (Figure A-3.10) Stop when you feel tension and wait for a release. Continue over the edge of scapula.

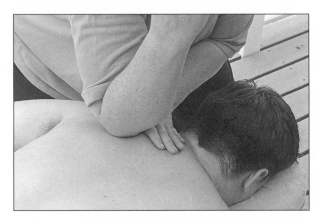

Figure A-3.9. Linear friction of tricep and supraspinatus

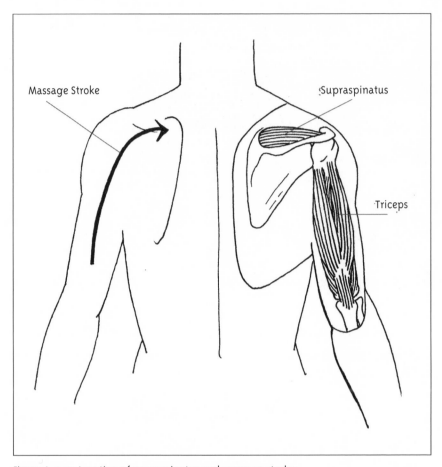

Figure A-3.10. Location of supraspinatus and massage stroke

Perform linear friction over infraspinatus. (Figure A-3.11) Start above elbow; glide up to acromion process, over mid-scapula and medial border of scapula. (Figure A-3.12)

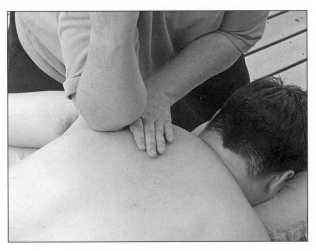

Figure A-3.11. Linear friction of infraspinatus

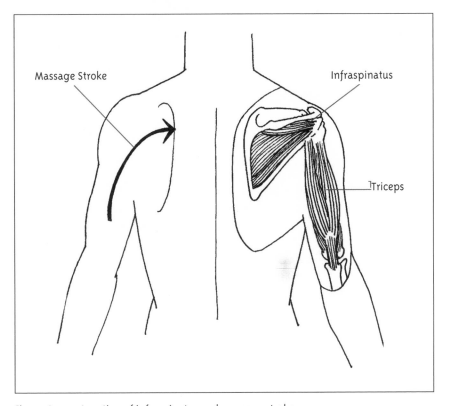

Figure A-3.12. Location of infraspinatus and massage stroke

Linear friction over teres minor. (Figure A-3.13) Start at elbow; glide up to acromion process and down inferior border of scapula to the inferior medial border. (Figure A-3.14)

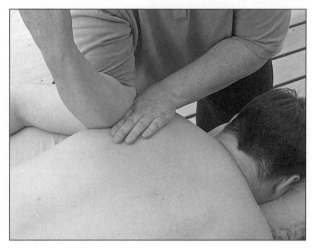

Figure A-3.13. Linear friction of teres minor

Move to the client's right side and perform cross-fiber friction on left erector spinae. Position your thumbs or knuckles just below the seventh cervical vertebra. Support your thumbs with loosely closed fists. Let your thumbs sink in to the lamina groove while standing on your tiptoes, then direct pressure away from spine (and yourself) as you flatten your feet. (Figure A-3.15) Use a short, scooping action. When you feel tightness, try to hold that spot and wait for the muscle to relax and roll beneath your thumbs. Try not to let the muscle "twang" by abruptly passing over it. Count the three long erector spinae muscles as you pass over them: the spinalis, longissimus, and iliocostalis. (Figure A-3.16) The spinalis courses right next to the spine, but only in the upper half of the back. Stop your stroke after you cross the iliocostalis. Continue down to superior border of the sacrum.

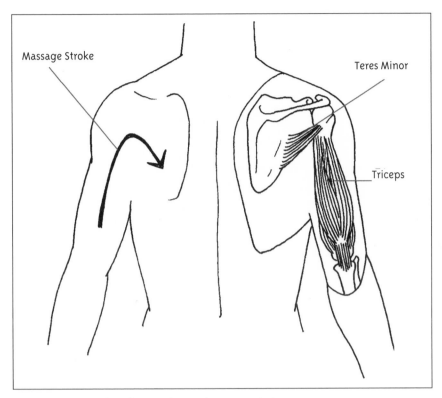

Figure A-3.14. Location of teres minor and massage stroke

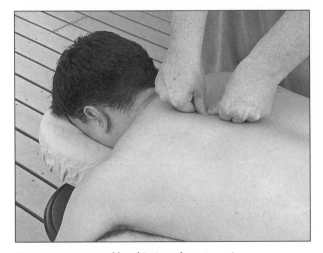

Figure A-3.15. Cross-fiber friction of erector spinae

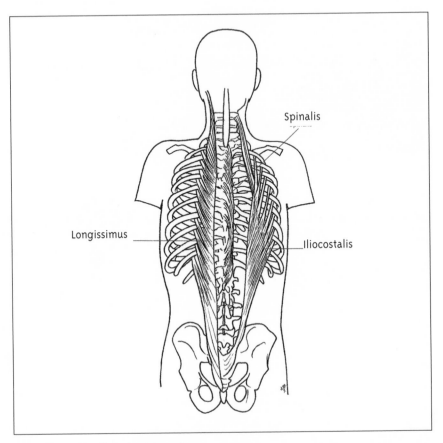

Figure A-3.16. Location of erector spinae

Position your thumbs just below the seventh cervical vertebra again. Stagger thumbs by rotating your body to a forty-five-degree angle to the table. Be sure to support your thumbs with loosely closed fists. (Figure A-3.17) This will address the important multifidi. (Figure A-3.18) Numerous studies have shown that many types of back pain sufferers have irregularities in the multifidi, regardless of the condition of the spine (Johnson, 2002). Begin on your tiptoes, just as you did with the erector spinae. Allow your thumbs to sink in, and then direct pressure away from the spine at a forty-five-degree angle, as you flatten your feet. Try not to just roll over tight multifidi; instead, hold pressure and wait for a release.

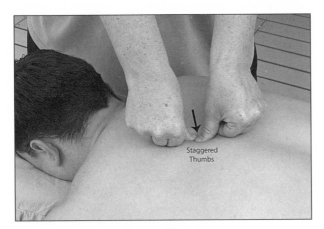

Figure A-3.17. Linear friction of multifidi

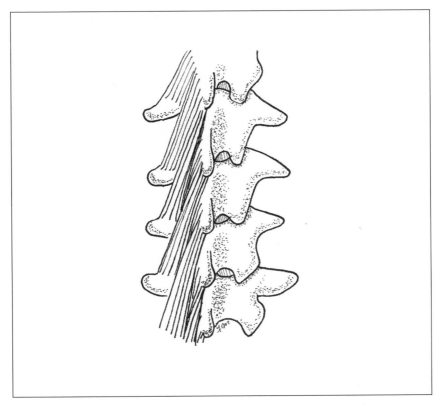

Figure A-3.18. Location of multifidi

Use some petrissage to "make nice," as our teacher Amon would say. Go to the head of the table, position both palms on upper traps on either side of the spine and slide down along spine to PSIS, back up the sides of body, and finish stroke by coming around shoulders to the base of skull. Repeat all steps on right side of back and right shoulder.

T2—**Lower Extremity (LE) Work**. Begin with effleurage to spread the oil from ankle to hip. Progress to petrissage from the client's ankle to buttock. Be sure to watch body mechanics by bending your knees, straightening your back, and shifting your weight from side to side. Use your whole body rather than just your arms. (Figure A-3.19)

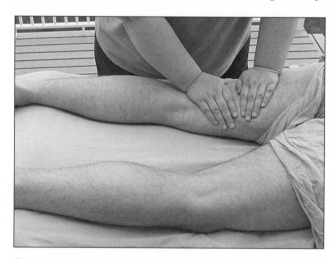

Figure A-3.19. Lower extremity petrissage

Tell your client that you will be doing several stretches. Ask him to relax his leg as much as possible, so you can do the passive stretches. Bring the ankle off the table, so the calf is at a ninety-degree angle. Cradle the front of the client's ankle with your inferior hand (the hand nearest foot of bed) shaped in a "C." Gently squeeze the Achilles tendon with your other hand. (Figure A-3.20) Rock the foot up and down in a teeter-totter fashion to massage the Achilles tendon.

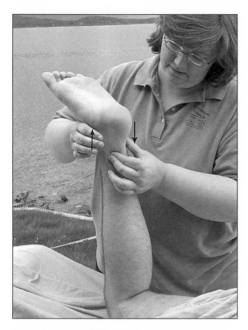

Figure A-3.20. Achilles tendon massage

Continue to hold the ankle at a ninety-degree angle with the same hand. Place your superior hand on the sacrum. This is your "mother hand" to feel for any signal that the stretch is uncomfortable. Jostle leg in a gentle circular pattern to reduce muscle guarding. Bring the foot across the body, toward the opposite hip, to stretch the vastus lateralis. (Figure A-3.21) Slide your hand holding the ankle to the middle of the client's foot to extend the ankle. Move slowly. Do not force this stretch past what is a natural stopping point.

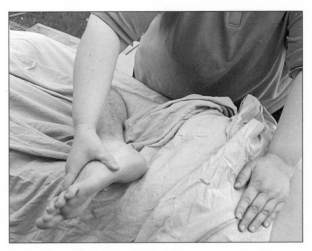

Figure A-3.21. Vastus lateralis stretch

Bring client's leg back to ninety-degree angle and jostle again to reduce muscle guarding. Bring client's foot toward ipsilateral buttock to stretch the quadriceps. (Figure A-3.22) Again, use slow movement and intuition to find the stopping point.

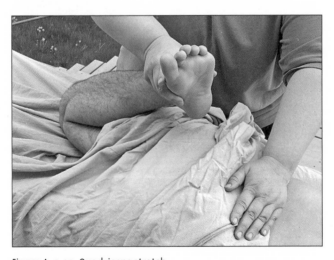

Figure A-3.22. Quadriceps stretch

Bring client's leg back to neutral ninety-degree angle. Keep your mother hand on the sacrum. Abduct client's foot away from midline as far as it will go without forcing it. Gently move foot superiorly toward hip to stretch the piriformis. (Figure A-3.23)

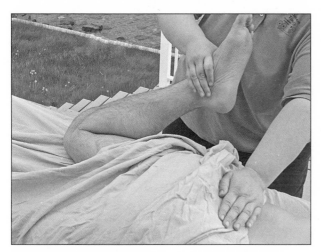

Figure A-3.23. Piriformis stretch

Bring foot back to neutral position at ninety-degree angle. Jostle gently. Lift client's leg off table to slide your inferior hand under the client's knee. Place your superior hand on the sacrum. Ask client to take in a deep breath and let it out slowly. As the client exhales, lift the knee and lower extremity off table to stretch the psoas and iliacus muscles. It is very important that the client exhales during this stretch. This shiatsu stretch is called "fisherman's cast." (Figure A-3.24) Note that T1 will coordinate a linear stroke up the erector spinae muscles to enhance the stretching effect.

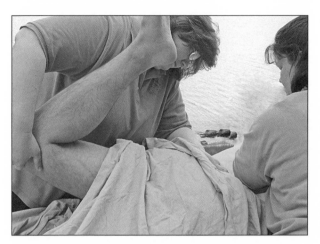

Figure A-3.24. Psoas and iliacus stretch

Bring client's thigh back down to the table, keeping the lower leg at a ninety-degree angle. Place your inferior forearm on the client's foot. Relax your forearm and hand. Lean your body weight into the client's foot, pushing his lower leg toward his buttock. Try to keep the client's foot parallel to table. This flexes the tibialis anterior and stretches the gastrocnemius and the rest of posterior calf muscles, as well as the quadriceps. (Figure A-3.25)

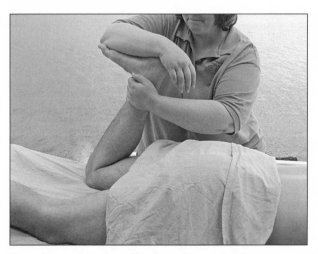

Figure A-3.25. Posterior calf and quadriceps stretch

Reposition lower extremity on table. Perform ankle to buttock effleurage and back down to ankle. Perform deep petrissage on posterior calf. (Figure A-3.26)

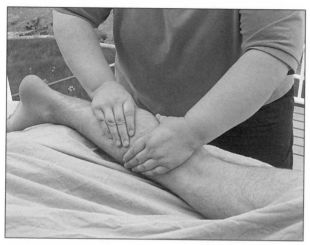

Figure A-3.26. Deep petrissage of posterior calf

Perform linear friction of gastrocnemius with thumbs (supported with loosely closed fist). (Figure A-3.27) Not much pressure is required for this as the calf is usually tender.

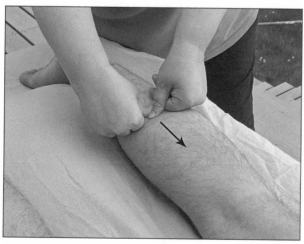

Figure A-3.27. Linear friction of gastrocnemius

Perform deep petrissage on posterior, medial, and lateral thigh. Continue deep petrissage to buttock, with particular attention to the posterior inferior iliac spine and greater trochanter areas. Use superior forearm to perform circular friction on hamstrings and iliotibial band from knee to greater trochanter. (Figures A-3.28 and A-3.29)

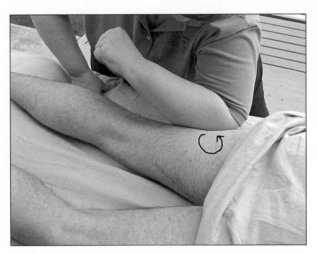

Figure A-3.28. Circular friction on TFL and iliotibial band

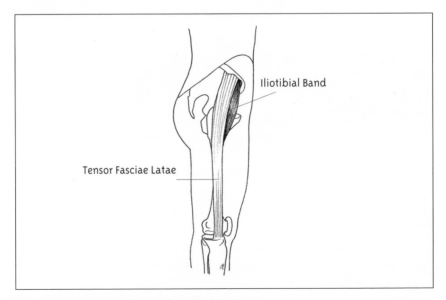

Figure A-3.29. Location of TFL and iliotibial band

Lean in with forearm just above lateral knee and slowly glide up iliotibial band to greater trochanter to perform linear friction. (Figure A-3.30)

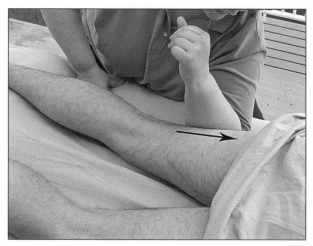

Figure A-3.30. Linear friction of TFL and iliotibial band

Just above the greater trochanter, plant your elbow on table and "windshield wiper" the tensor fasciae latae. (Figure A-3.31)

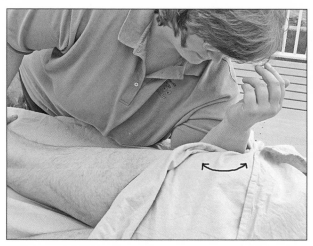

Figure A-3.31. "Windshield wiper" of tensor fasciae latae

Lean in with forearm just above posterior knee and slowly glide up hamstrings to greater trochanter. (Figure A-3.32) Continue over gluteals and slide forearm back down to knee.

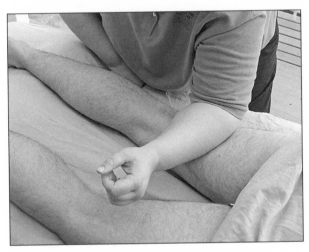

Figure A-3.32. Linear friction on hamstrings

Place closed fist with heel of hand on medial thigh just above knee. Move in a circular pattern, then lean in and glide straight up the adductors for linear friction. (Figure A-3.33) Monitor your pressure on client tolerance and muscle response.

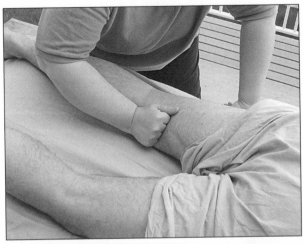

Figure A-3.33. Linear friction of adductors

Continue up over the gluteals. Place the tip of your elbow at the sacroiliac joint. Adjust draping to perform on bare skin. Move down medial border of sacrum to soften the gluteus maximus. (Figure A-3.34) Be careful not to use too much pressure, as this could impinge the sciatic nerve. Ask the client to tell you if he begins to feel numbness or tingling.

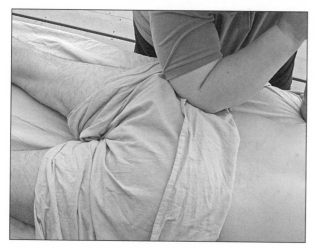

Figure A-3.34. Deep work on gluteus maximus

Release pressure at inferior sacrum and bring forearm back up over gluteals. Place tip of elbow at lateral edge of iliac crest. Use your body weight to slowly sink your elbow tip through the gluteals and glide inferiorly to contact the insertion sites of the deep lateral hip rotators. (Figure A-3.35) If the piriformis or other rotators feel tight, stop and wait for the muscle to melt. (Figure A-3.36) Then continue your stroke to the inferior edge of the gluteus maximus. Release pressure and move forearm in circular motion over gluteals to soothe the area.

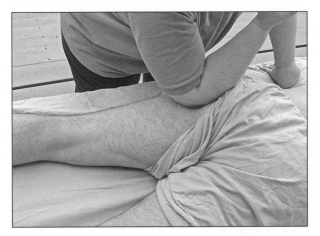

Figure A-3.35. Working insertion sites of the deep hip rotators

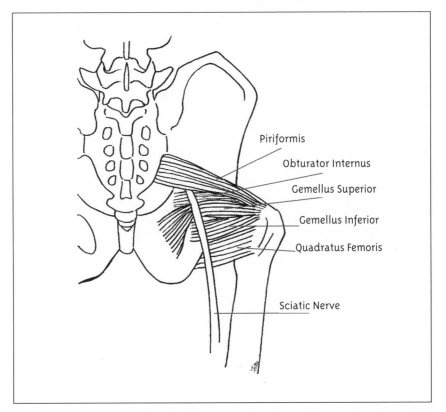

Figure A-3.36. Location of deep lateral hip rotators

Continue circular friction with forearm down the thigh and calf. Perform a long effleurage stroke from ankle to iliac crest. Spread fingers. Move arms quickly back and forth while gliding down to ankle. This creates a fine vibration to sedate the nervous system. (Figure A-3.37)

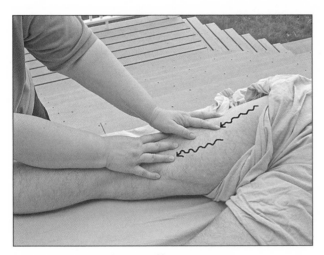

Figure A-3.37. Fine vibration of lower extremity

Replace draping over lower extremity. Perform compressions from iliac crest to foot. (Figure A-3.38)

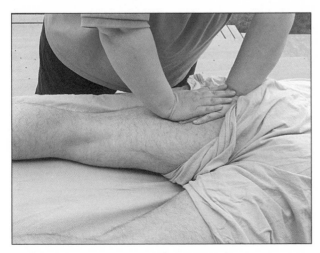

Figure A-3.38. Compressions on lower extremity

Use heel of superior hand in three small circular patterns at medial border of mid sacrum to loosen and soften tissue. (Figure A-3.39)

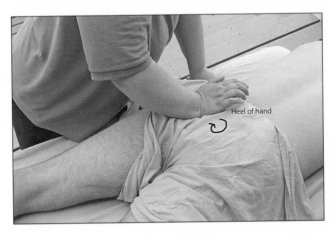

Figure A-3.39. Circular motion at mid sacrum

Use heel of inferior hand and repeat circular motion between posterior inferior iliac spine (sitz bone) and greater trochanter. (Figure A-3.40)

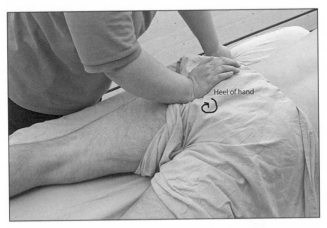

Figure A-3.40. Circular motion near greater trochanter

Repeat all T2 steps with left leg.

4. SYNCHRONOUS—SEQUENCE TO FINISH POSTERIOR SIDE OF BODY

T1 and T2 position inferior forearms on either side of the body at iliac crest (PSIS). Both therapists apply pressure near spine and down PSIS in a sawing motion for transverse friction of quadratus lumborum. (Figure A-4.1)

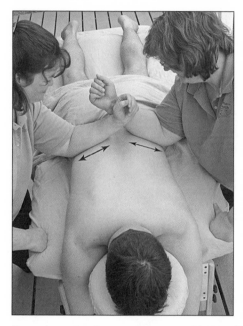

Figure A-4.1. *Synchronous transverse friction of quadratus lumborum*

Use forearms in a large circular motion up the sides of back. Glide over shoulder and down triceps. Bring forearms back to the axilla and glide down latissimus dorsi to iliac crest. (Figure A-4.2)

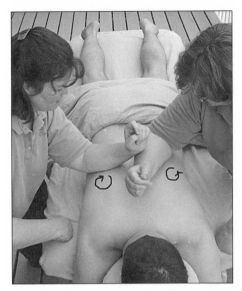

Figure A-4.2. *Synchronous circular friction on back*

Glide elbow tips up either side of the spine for linear friction on erector spinae from sacrum to top of scapula. (Figure A-4.3) Be careful to stay off the spinous processes.

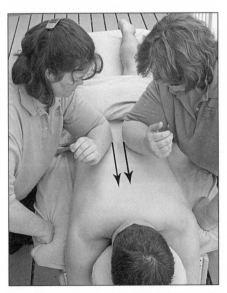

Figure A-4.3. *Synchronous linear friction of erectors*

Slide forearms to side of body and lean your body weight in gently. Stroke down the latissimus dorsi. (Figure A-4.4) You may wish to repeat the linear friction of erectors and synchronous latissimus dorsi stroke. Clients appreciate these movements.

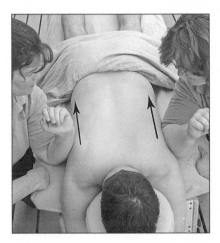

Figure A-4.4. *Synchronous latissimus dorsi stroke*

When the PSIS is reached, begin synchronous petrissage strokes up the back. (Figure A-4.5) Rock your body weight and time your movement with your fellow therapist to assist in synchronizing your petrissage.

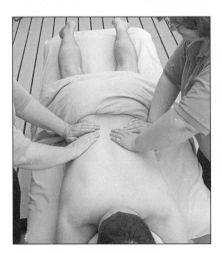

Figure A-4.5. *Synchronous back petrissage*

When the upper trapezius is reached, relax muscle with deep petrissage. Hook fingertips of both hands around the superior border of upper trapezius and pull downward to stretch the upper trapezius. (Figure A-4.6)

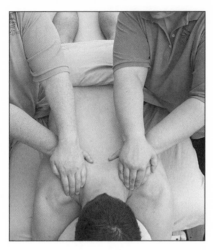

Figure A-4.6. *Upper trapezius stretch*

Loosen your grip and move hands quickly back and forth to create vibratory effect. Continue from upper trapezius to sacrum. (Figure A-4.7) Keep wrists and fingers straight. Move elbows to create short back and forth motion.

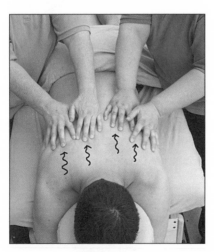

Figure A-4.7. *Synchronous back vibration*

Stretch out lower back and quadratus lumborum by placing one forearm on iliac crest (PSIS) and the other forearm just below the scapula. (Figure A-4.8) Press down and stretch muscle by moving forearms apart.

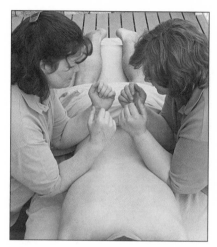

Figure A-4.8. *Lower back stretch*

Reposition draping over back. Perform synchronous compressions from upper back to feet. Remember to ask client to take in a deep breath and exhale slowly. Compress during exhalation and move hand position during inhalation. (Figure A-4.9)

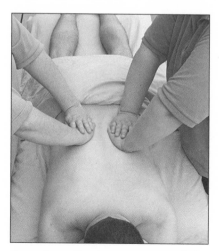

Figure A-4.9. *Synchronous compressions*

Finish posterior side of body by lightly brushing down sides of body from head to toe with fingertips. (Figure A-4.10) This brings negative energy out the feet and resets the parasympathetic nervous system.

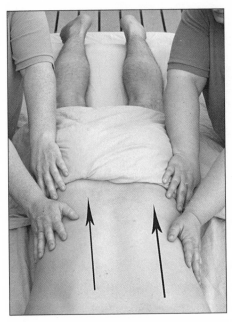

Figure A-4.10. *Brushing down sides of body*

Hold both sides of draping. Tell the client that you have reached the turning point. Ask him to scoot down toward the foot of the table and then turn over onto his back.

Steps 5–14. Supine Lower Extremities

5. SYNCHRONOUS—SEQUENCE TO BEGIN WORK ON SUPINE LOWER EXTREMITIES

T1 and T2—Perform compressions up the lower extremities from ankle to hip to follow the direction of yin energy flow. The yin meridians flow up the body on the anterior body and soft, inner surfaces of the limbs. (Figure A-5.1)

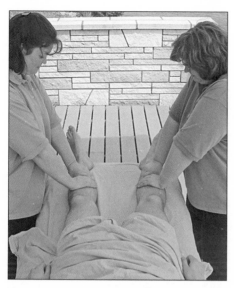

Figure A-5.1. *Compressing up lower extremities*

T1 and T2—Brush down ("apana vayu") from hip to ankle. (Figure A-5.2) This stroke is in the opposite direction of yin energy to bring negative energy away from the center of the body and out the feet.

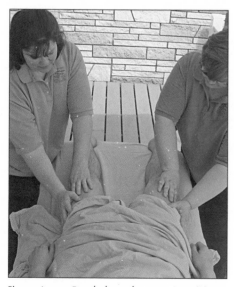

Figure A-5.2. *Brush down lower extremities*

Both therapists grasp the side of sheet and place between the client's legs. Each therapist separately takes hold of the sheet from under the client's knee and brings it up to tuck under client's hip, creating a "diaper" effect. (Figure A-5.3)

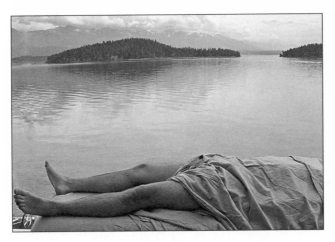

Figure A-5.3. *Draping technique for lower extremity work*

Both therapists begin near ankle with synchronous effleurage to spread lotion. Then petrissage strokes are performed synchronously from ankle to hip and back down to the ankle. Coordinating the rocking movements created by shifting weight from superior leg to inferior leg can easily synchronize these strokes.

6. ASYNCHRONOUS—T1 BENT KNEE CALF WORK, T2 STRAIGHT LEG THIGH WORK

T1—Bend left knee up and sit gently on client's foot to stabilize his leg. With hands on each side of the calf and fingers reaching to opposite side of calf, move calf to right with right hand and to left with left hand. Alternate hands in a wringing motion for transverse friction of posterior calf muscles. (Figure A-6.1)

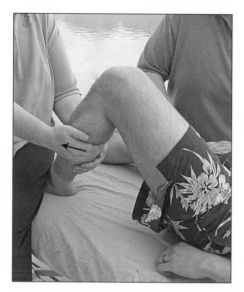

Figure A-6.1. Transverse friction of posterior calf muscles

With fingertips aligned in center of upper posterior calf, gently pull fingertips apart to separate the two heads of the gastrocnemeus muscle. (Figures A-6.2 and A-6.3)

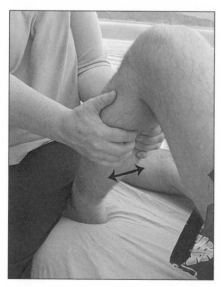

Figure A-6.2. Separating the heads of the gastrocnemius

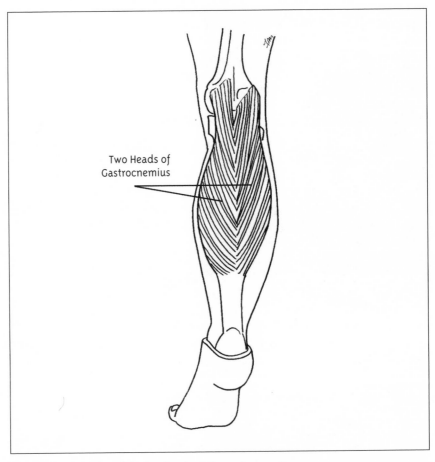

Figure A-6.3. Location of the two heads of the gastrocnemius

Lace fingers together and place on top of thigh as near to the groin as is comfortable for both you and your client. Press in and glide hands toward the knee to perform linear friction of the quadriceps. (Figure A-6.4) Repeat on inner thigh adductors (Figure A-6.5) and outer thigh vastus lateralis, tensor fasciae latae, and iliotibial band. (Figure A-6.6)

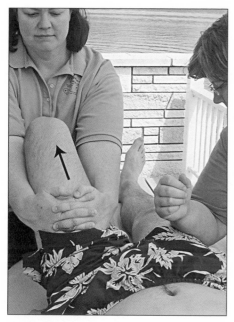

Figure A-6.4. Linear friction of the quadriceps

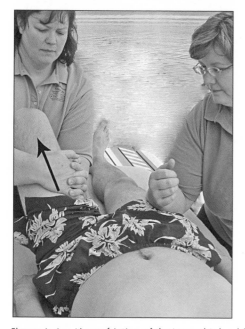

Figure A-6.5. Linear friction of the inner thigh adductors

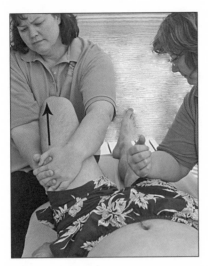

Figure A-6.6. Linear friction of the outer thigh muscles

Straighten leg as you stand from seated position. Perform soothing petrissage on entire lower extremity.

T2—Perform petrissage of right thigh. Then use forearm to perform circular (Figure A-6.7) and transverse "sawing" friction to lateral thigh muscles: vastus lateralis, tensor fasciae latae, and iliotibial band. (Figure A-6.8)

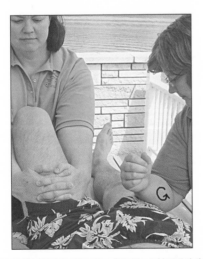

Figure A-6.7. Circular friction of lateral thigh muscles

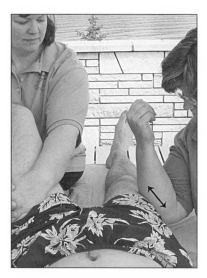

Figure A-6.8. Transverse friction of lateral thigh muscles

Beginning just above the knee, press forearm in and glide up to greater trochanter for linear friction of the lateral thigh muscles. (Figure A-6.9) Envision a lengthening response. These muscles are often tight and can be the cause of hip and low back pain.

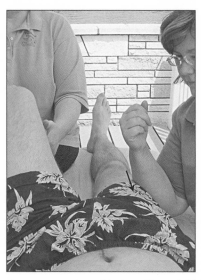

Figure A-6.9. Linear friction of lateral thigh muscle

Slide your forearm or closed fist (use pads of back of fingers) to inner thigh. Move in slow circles from knee to the inner thigh as far as is comfortable for you and your client. (Figure A-6.10)

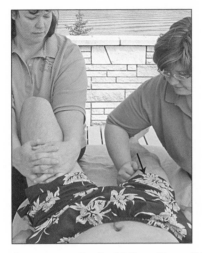

Figure A-6.10. Circular friction of inner thigh adductors

Use forearm or closed fist to glide from knee to as close to the groin as is comfortable for linear friction of adductors. (Figure A-6.11)

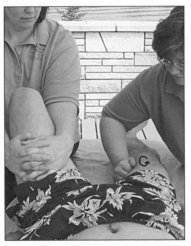

Figure A-6.11. Linear friction of adductors

Petrissage entire lower extremity.

7. SYNCHRONOUS—LOWER EXTREMITY CONNECTING STROKE

T1 and T2 glide with flat palms from ankle to hip and back down. (Figure A-7.1)

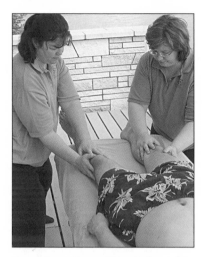

Figure A-7.1. *Connecting stroke on lower extremities*

8. ASYNCHRONOUS—T1 STRAIGHT-LEG THIGH WORK, T2 BENT-KNEE CALF WORK

T1—Perform petrissage of left thigh. Then use forearm to perform circular (Figure A-8.1) and transverse "sawing" friction to lateral thigh muscles: vastus lateralis, tensor fasciae latae, and iliotibial band. (Figure A-8.2)

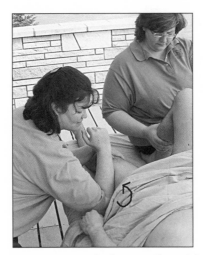

Figure A-8.1. Circular friction of lateral thigh muscles

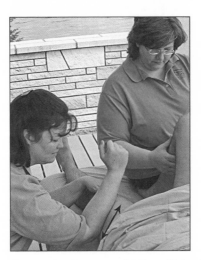

Figure A-8.2. Transverse friction of lateral thigh muscles

Beginning just above the knee, press forearm in and glide up to greater trochanter for linear friction of the lateral thigh muscles. (Figure A-8.3) Envision a lengthening response. These muscles are often tight and can be the cause of hip and low back pain.

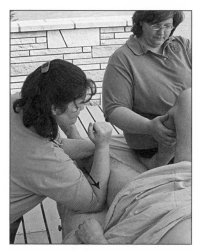

Figure A-8.3. Linear friction of lateral thigh muscles

Slide your forearm or closed fist (use pads of back of fingers) to inner thigh. (Figure A-8.4) Move in slow circles from knee to the inner thigh as far as is comfortable for you and your client.

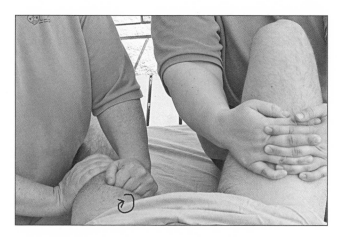

Figure A-8.4. Circular friction of inner thigh adductors

Use forearm or closed fist to glide from medial knee to as close to the groin as is comfortable for linear friction of adductors. (Figure A-8.5)

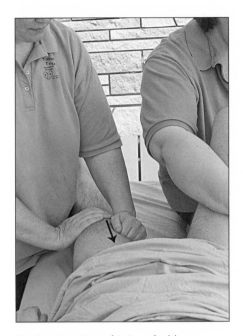

Figure A-8.5. Linear friction of adductors

Petrissage entire lower extremity.

T2—Bend left knee up and sit gently on client's foot to stabilize his leg. With hands on each side of the calf and fingers reaching to opposite side of calf, move calf to right with right hand and to left with left hand. Alternate hands in a wringing motion for transverse friction of posterior calf muscles. (Figure A-8.6)

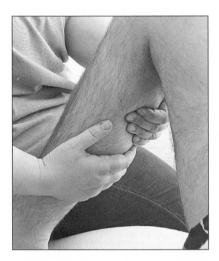

Figure A-8.6. Transverse friction of posterior calf muscles

With fingertips aligned in center of upper posterior calf, gently pull fingertips apart to separate the two heads of the gastrocnemeus muscle. (Figure A-8.7)

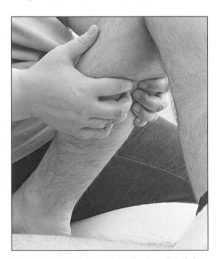

Figure A-8.7. Separating the heads of the gastrocnemius

Interlock fingers together and place on top of anterior thigh as near to the groin as is comfortable for both you and your client. Press in and glide hands toward the knee to perform linear friction of the quadriceps.

(Figure A-8.8) Repeat on inner thigh adductors (Figure A-8.9) and outer thigh vastus lateralis, tensor fasciae latae, and iliotibial band. (Figure A-8.10)

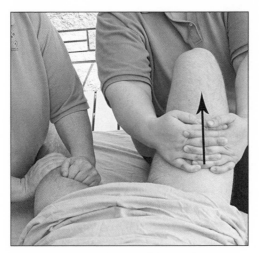

Figure A-8.8. Linear friction of the quadriceps

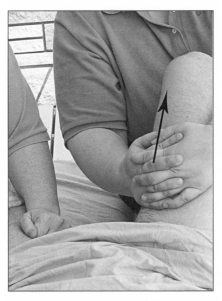

Figure A-8.9. Linear friction of the inner thigh adductors

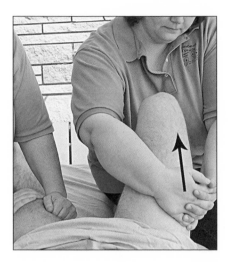

Figure A-8.10. Linear friction of the outer thigh muscles

Straighten leg as you stand from seated position. Perform soothing petrissage on entire lower extremity.

9. SYNCHRONOUS—LOWER EXTREMITY CONNECTING STROKE

T1 and T2 glide with flat palms from ankle to hip and back down. (Figure A-9.1)

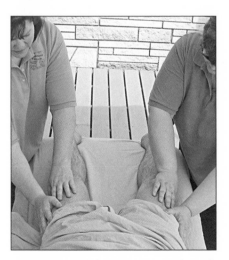

Figure A-9.1. *Simple connecting stroke on lower extremities*

10. ASYNCHRONOUS—T1 PERFORMS LOWER EXTREMITY STRETCHES, T2 PERFORMS CALF WORK

T1—Cup left hand around client's left heel. Support client's knee with right hand. Slowly bend knee while raising foot to perform hamstrings stretch. Do not force this passive stretch. (Figure A-10.1)

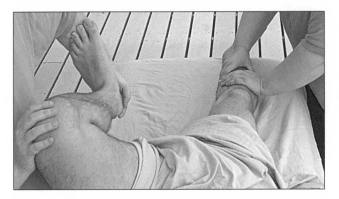

Figure A-10.1. Hamstrings stretch

Release stretch and rotate hip in circular fashion once or twice. Let go of heel and move your left hand to client's knee. Place right mother hand on client's shoulder. Push knee across client's body. Make sure the client's lower back remains on table. This stretches the lateral thigh muscles. (Figure A-10.2)

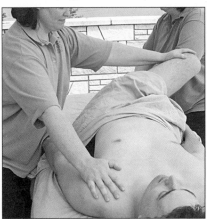

Figure A-10.2. Lateral thigh stretch

Release stretch. Reposition draping. Cup left hand around heel again and place right hand on inside of knee. Guide knee away from midline, while allowing heel to move medially to stretch inner thigh adductors. (Figure A-10.3) Be careful to reposition the draping. You may wish to guide the stretch by pulling the sheet tight around inner thigh. Push down gently on medial knee to increase stretch slightly.

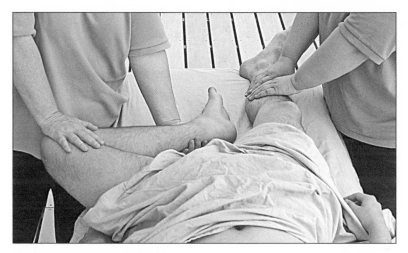

Figure A-10.3. Inner thigh stretch

Keep your left hand cupped around left heel. Gently place right mother hand on top of client's patella. Be careful not to exert any pressure on the patella during this stretch. Slowly raise client's straight lower extremity to stretch posterior calf muscles. (Figure A-10.4)

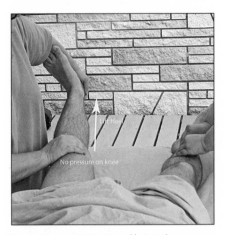

Figure A-10.4. Posterior calf stretch

Perform "dragon's mouth" lower leg stretches by spreading your right thumb from fingers and pressing down with right hand near client's left knee, while pushing the client's ball of foot toward knee. The dorsiflexion is then released and right hand moves down several inches. In a teeter-totter fashion, the foot is dorsiflexed again, while pressing down with "dragon's mouth." Release and move right hand down several inches. Repeat several times until ankle is reached. (Figure A-10.5)

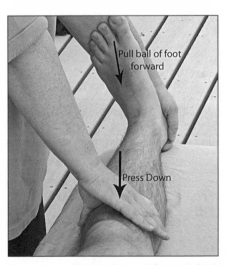

Figure A-10.5. "Dragon's mouth" stretch for lower leg

T2—Perform deep petrissage before beginning deep tissue. Feel the client's shinbone (tibia). Place thumbs or knuckles on tibia several inches above ankle. Allow your thumbs or knuckles to slide laterally into the indentation between the tibia and the extensor digitorum longus. Press into muscle, direct pressure laterally, and wait for a release. (Figure A-10.6) Move thumbs or knuckles up a couple inches and repeat until knee is reached. Be sure to support your thumbs with a closed fist. This affects the tibialis anterior as well.

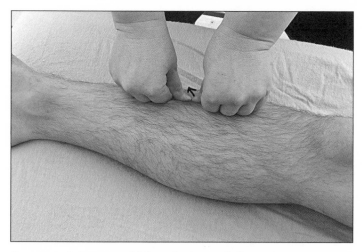

Figure A-10.6. Transverse friction of extensor digitorum longus

Perform linear friction of extensor digitorum longus using supported thumbs or elbow. Guide your elbow between the thumb and index finger of your opposite hand. Begin several inches above ankle and glide slowly up to just below the knee. (Figure A-10.7)

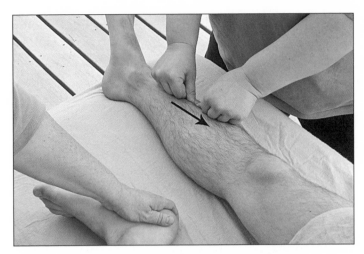

Figure A-10.7. Linear friction of the extensor digitorum longus

II. SYNCHRONOUS—LOWER EXTREMITY CONNECTING STROKE

T1 and T2 glide with flat palms from ankle to hip and back down. (Figure A-11.1)

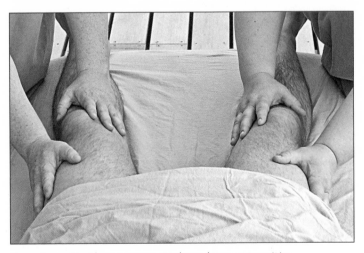

Figure A-11.1. *Simple connecting stroke on lower extremities*

12. ASYNCHRONOUS—T1 PERFORMS CALF WORK, T2 PERFORMS LOWER EXTREMITY STRETCHES

T1—Perform deep petrissage before beginning deep tissue. Feel the client's shinbone. Place thumbs or knuckles on tibia several inches above ankle. Allow your thumbs or knuckles to slide laterally into the indentation between the tibia and the extensor digitorum longus. Press into muscle, direct pressure laterally, and wait for a release. (Figure A-12.1) Move thumbs or knuckles up a couple inches and repeat until knee is reached. This affects the tibialis anterior as well.

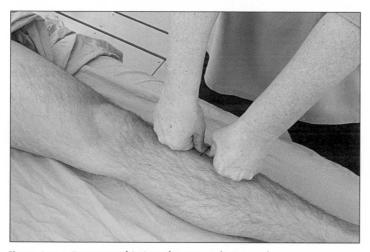

Figure A-12.1. Transverse friction of extensor digitorum longus

Perform linear friction of extensor digitorum longus using supported thumbs or elbow. Guide your elbow between the thumb and index finger of your opposite hand. Begin several inches above ankle and glide slowly up to just below the knee. (Figure A-12.2)

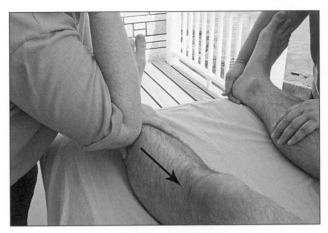

Figure A-12.2. Linear friction of the extensor digitorum longus

T2—Cup right hand around the client's right heel. Support the client's knee with your left hand. Slowly bend knee while raising foot to perform hamstrings stretch. Do not force this passive stretch. (Figure A-12.3)

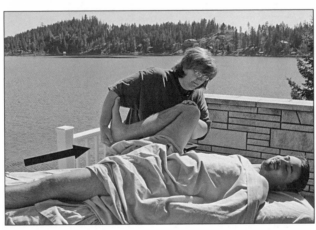

Figure A-12.3. Hamstrings stretch

Release stretch and rotate hip in circular fashion once or twice. Let go of heel and move your right hand to client's knee. Place left mother hand on client's shoulder. Push knee across client's body. Make sure the client's lower back remains on table. This stretches the lateral thigh muscles. (Figure A-12.4)

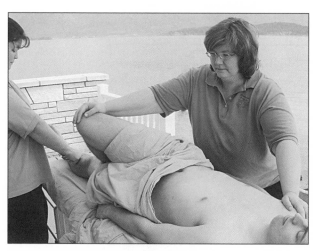

Figure A-12.4. Lateral thigh stretch

Release stretch. Reposition draping. Cup right hand around heel again and place left hand on inside of knee. Guide knee away from midline while allowing heel to move medially to stretch inner thigh adductors. (Figure A-12.5) Be careful to reposition the draping. You may wish to guide the stretch by pulling the sheet tight around inner thigh. Push down gently on medial knee to increase stretch slightly.

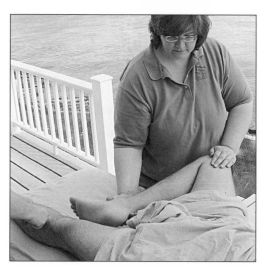

Figure A-12.5. Inner thigh stretch

Keep your right hand cupped around right heel. Gently place left mother hand on top of the client's patella. Be careful not to exert any pressure on the patella during this stretch. Slowly raise client's straight lower extremity to stretch posterior calf muscles. (Figure A-12.6)

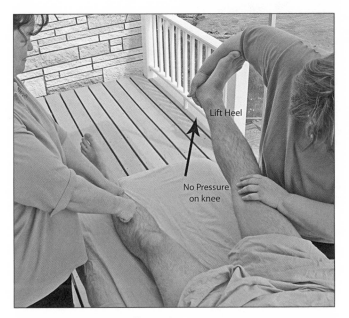

Figure A-12.6. Posterior calf stretch

Perform "dragon's mouth" lower leg stretches by spreading your left thumb from fingers and pressing down with left hand near client's right knee, while pushing the client's ball of foot toward knee. The dorsiflexion is then released and left hand moves down several inches. In a teeter-totter fashion, the foot is dorsiflexed again, while pressing down with "dragon's mouth." Release and move left hand down several inches. Repeat several times until ankle is reached. (Figure A-12.7)

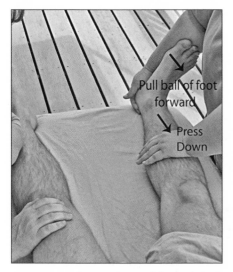

Figure A-12.7. "Dragon's mouth" stretch for lower leg

13. SYNCHRONOUS—LOWER EXTREMITY CONNECTING STROKE

T1 and T2 glide with flat palms from ankle to hip and back down. (Figure A-13.1)

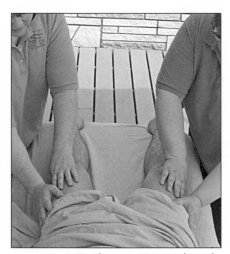

Figure A-13.1. *Simple connecting stroke on lower extremities*

Both therapists replace sheet to cover client's lower extremities.

14. SYNCHRONOUS—SEQUENCE TO FINISH LOWER EXTREMITY

T1 and T2—Palm up the lower extremities from ankle to hip, following the yin meridians. (Figure A-14.1)

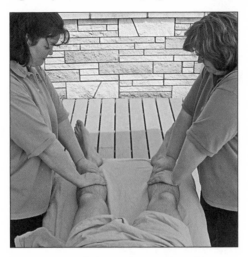

Figure A-14.1. *Palming up lower extremities*

T1 and T2—Brush down (apana vayu stroke) lower extremities. (Figure A-14.2)

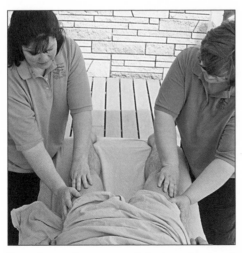

Figure A-14.2. *Apana vayu stoke down lower extremities*

Steps 15–19. Upper Extremities

15. SYNCHRONOUS—UPPER EXTREMITY

T1 and T2 lightly brush down arms to let client know your will be massaging his arms next. Grasp the side of sheet and place between client's torso and arm. Lift arm off table and bring sheet under arm in usual draping fashion. (Figure A-15.1)

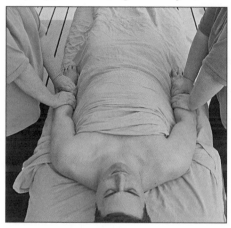

Figure A-15.1. *Upper extremity draping*

T1 and T2 perform bilateral palming compressions up the yin meridians from wrist to shoulder. (Figure A-15.2)

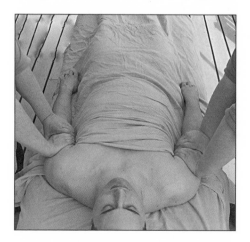

Figure A-15.2. *Synchronized palming up upper extremity*

Glide back down to fingertips with synchronized apana vayu stroke. (Figure A-15.3)

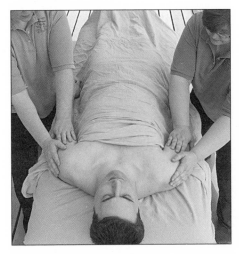

Figure A-15.3. *Synchronized apana vayu stroke*

Begin near wrist with effleurage up arm to spread lubricant. Perform synchronous petrissage from wrist to shoulder and back down to wrist. Coordinate the rocking movements created by shifting weight from superior leg to inferior leg to help to synchronize these strokes. (Figure A-15.4)

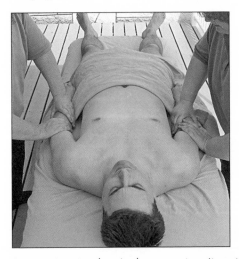

Figure A-15.4. *Synchronized upper extremity petrissage*

T1 and T2 slide one hand under client's hand and the other on top of client's hand to lift hand for synchronized hand massage. Change your stance to face the head of table. Place hands on either side of the wrist. Jostle gently to mobilize wrist joint. Rotate wrist in bicycle fashion. (Figure A-15.5)

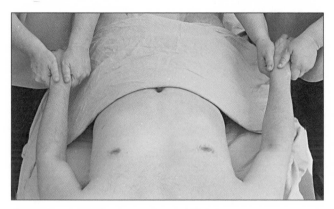

Figure A-15.5. *Synchronous wrist mobilization*

Slide hands out to first knuckles of client's hands. Support hand with the fingers of both of your hands. Place your thumbs between each large knuckle at the metacarpophalangeal joint. Apply pressure and stroke down toward wrist between each metacarpal to the carpal bones. (Figure A-15.6) Pay particular attention to the thumb metacarpal.

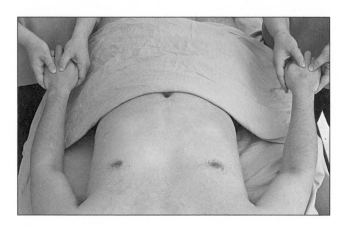

Figure A-15.6. *Linear strokes on dorsum of hands*

Invert client's hand, so palm is facing up. Place your little finger between the client's index and middle fingers. Place the little finger of your other hand between the client's ring and little fingers. Support the client's hand with your other fingers. (Figure A-15.7)

Move your little fingers gently apart to stretch client's hand.

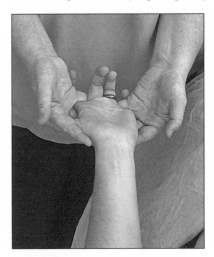

Figure A-15.7. *Hand stretch*

Press in at the center of the heel of client's palm with both thumbs. Glide to sides of hand to stretch palm muscles. Move toward fingers and repeat. Repeat to knuckles and back to heel of hand. (Figure A-15.8)

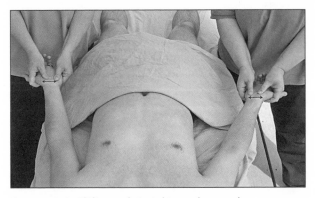

Figure A-15.8. *Gliding and stretching palm muscles*

Release stretch by removing your little fingers. Hold wrist with all fingers of both hands. Use thumbs for circular friction in palm of client's hands. (Figure A-15.9)

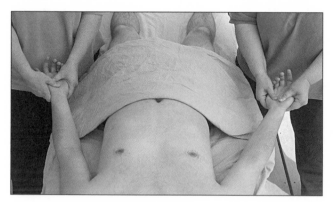

Figure A-15.9. *Circular friction in palm*

Turn client's hand palm down. Synchronously massage each digit from first knuckle out to tip beginning with the thumb and finishing with the little finger. (Figure A-15.10)

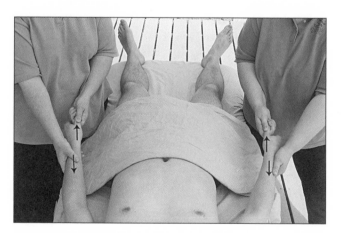

Figure A-15.10. *Synchronous digit massage*

16. ASYNCHRONOUS—T1 LEFT UPPER EXTREMITY DEEP TISSUE, T2 RIGHT UPPER EXTREMITY STRETCHES

T1—Use forearm or thumbs to perform circular friction of wrist extensor muscles in forearm. Begin with forearm or both thumbs in center of client's forearm just above wrist. Create small circles, while moving slowly up to elbow. (Figure A-16.1)

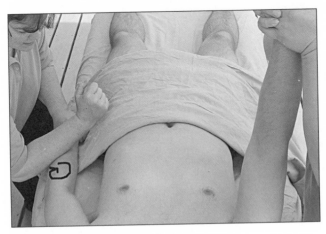

Figure A-16.1. Circular friction of wrist extensors

Turn your palm down and close your fist. Place the middle knuckles of your fingers on the elbow. Keep your wrist straight as you use short strokes on the common extensor tendon origin at lateral epicondyle of humerus with client's palm down. (Figure A-16.2)

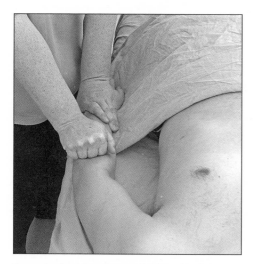

Figure A-16.2. Deep tissue of extensor origin

Turn client's palm up. Use short strokes with your knuckles just below the client's anterior medial epicondyle of humerus. Repeat several times, moving slightly each time. This is the common origin of the major flexors of the wrist. (Figure A-16.3)

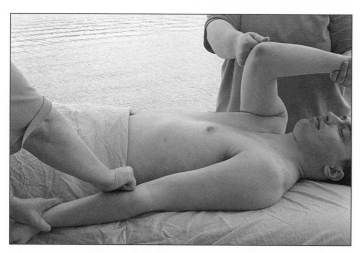

Figure A-16.3. Deep tissue of flexor origin

Soothe forearm with petrissage. Move to upper arm with continuous petrissage. (Figure A-16.4)

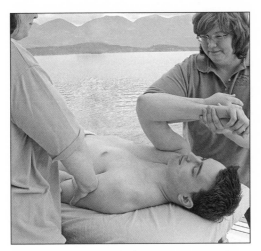

Figure A-16.4. Petrissage of upper arm

Assess if deep tissue is needed in upper arm. Apply as needed. Continue petrissage until T2 is ready for synchronous section.

T2—Grasp client's wrist and raise his arm straight up. Use both hands to gently pull arm upward to stretch shoulder muscles. This passive shiatsu stretch is called "reaching to heaven." (Figure A-16.5)

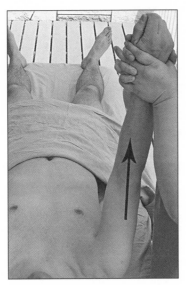

Figure A-16.5. "Reaching to heaven"

Release stretch. Let client's arm bend naturally. Lift wrist up and down in circular pattern to create "coffee grinder" joint play. (Figure A-16.6)

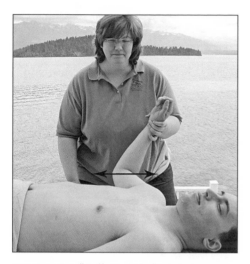

Figure A-16.6. "Coffee grinder" joint play

Hold wrist with inferior hand. Position client's arm in a ninety-degree angle. Interlock your superior elbow into client's elbow. (Figure A-16.7) Shift body weight backward to stretch upper arm and shoulder girdle. This passive shiatsu stretch is called "crane's embrace."

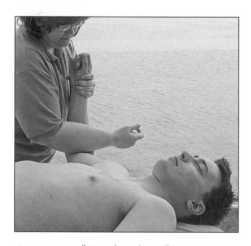

Figure A-16.7. "Crane's embrace"

Release stretch. Continue to hold client's wrist at ninety degrees with your inferior hand. Remove your elbow from client's elbow. Swing client's arm up so his forearm is parallel to the table and place your superior forearm against his forearm. Slowly push superior elbow toward the middle of the table, being careful to only stretch as far as comfortable for the client. (Figure A-16.8) This passive shiatsu stretch is called "fighter's pose."

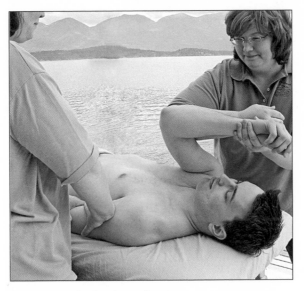

Figure A-16.8. "Fighter's pose"

Release stretch. Slowly straighten client's arm above his head and pull gently to stretch the triceps and shoulder muscles. (Figure A-16.9)

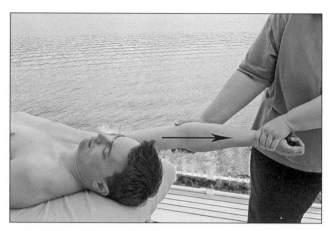

Figure A-16.9. Triceps stretch

Place client's arm back down at his side.

17. SYNCHRONOUS—UPPER EXTREMITY CONNECTING STROKE

T1 and T2 perform connective effleurage stroke. Use both palms beginning at wrist. Stroke upward synchronously to shoulder and back down to fingertips. (Figure A-17.1)

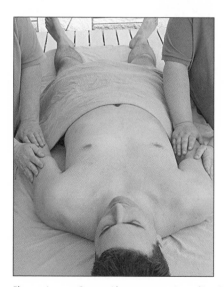

Figure A-17.1. *Connective upper extremity stroke*

Reposition client's arm at sides. Perform another synchronous effleurage stroke from wrist to shoulder and back down before beginning next asynchronous section.

18. ASYNCHRONOUS—T1 LEFT UPPER EXTREMITY STRETCHES, T2 RIGHT UPPER EXTREMITY DEEP TISSUE

T1—Grasp client's wrist and raise his arm straight up. Use both hands to gently pull arm upward to stretch shoulder muscles. This passive shiatsu stretch is called "reaching to heaven." (Figure A-18.1)

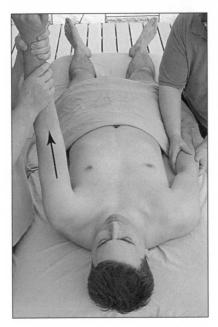

Figure A-18.1. "Reaching to heaven"

Release stretch. Let client's arm bend naturally. Lift wrist up and down in circular pattern to create "coffee grinder" joint play. (Figure A-18.2)

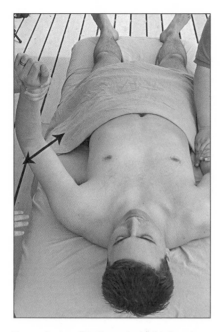

Figure A-18.2. "Coffee grinder" joint play

Hold wrist with inferior hand. Position client's arm in a ninety-degree angle. Interlock your superior elbow into client's elbow. (Figure A-18.3) Shift body weight backward to stretch upper arm and shoulder girdle. This passive shiatsu stretch is called "crane's embrace."

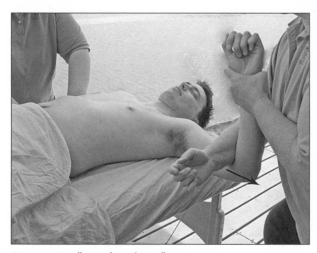

Figure A-18.3. "Crane's embrace"

Release stretch. Continue to hold client's wrist at ninety degrees with your inferior hand. Remove your elbow from client's elbow. Swing client's arm up so his forearm is parallel to the table and place your superior forearm against your client's forearm. Slowly push superior elbow toward the middle of the table, being careful to only stretch as far as is comfortable for the client. (Figure A-18.4) This passive shiatsu stretch is called "fighter's pose."

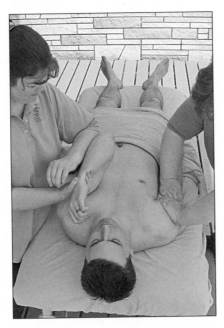

Figure A-18.4. "Fighter's pose"

Release stretch. Slowly straighten client's arm above his head and pull gently to stretch the triceps and shoulder muscles. (Figure A-18.5)

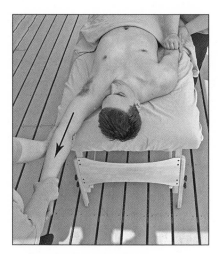

Figure A-18.5. Triceps stretch

Place client's arm back down at his side.

T2—Use forearm or thumbs to perform circular friction of wrist extensor muscles in forearm. (Figure A-18.6) Begin with forearm or both thumbs in center of client's forearm just above wrist. Create small circles while moving slowly up to elbow.

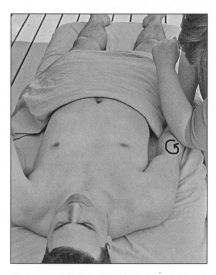

Figure A-18.6. Circular friction of wrist extensors

Turn your palm down and close your fist. Place the middle knuckles of your fingers on the elbow. Keep your wrist straight as you use short strokes on the common extensor tendon origin at lateral epicondyle of humerus with client's palm down. (Figure A-18.7)

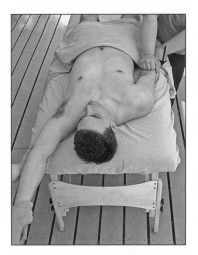

Figure A-18.7. Deep tissue of extensor origin

Turn client's palm up. Use short strokes with your knuckles just below the client's anterior medial epicondyle of humerus. Repeat several times, moving slightly each time. This is the common origin of the major flexors of the wrist. (Figure A-18.8)

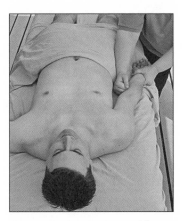

Figure A-18.8. Deep tissue of flexor origin

Soothe forearm with petrissage. Move to upper arm with continuous petrissage. (Figure A-18.9)

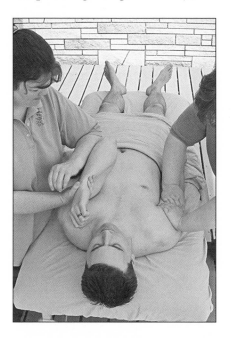

Figure A-18.9. Petrissage of upper arm

Assess if deep tissue is needed in upper arm. Apply as needed. Continue petrissage until T1 is ready for synchronous section.

19. SYNCHRONOUS—UPPER EXTREMITY FINISHING SEQUENCE

T1 and T2 perform effleurage stroke. Use both palms beginning at wrist. Stroke upward synchronously to shoulder and back down to fingertips. (Figure A-19.1)

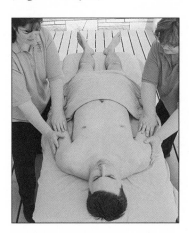

Figure A-19.1. *Connective upper extremity stroke*

Replace sheet over upper extremities. T1 and T2 perform bilateral palming compressions up the yin meridians from wrist to shoulder. (Figure A-19.2)

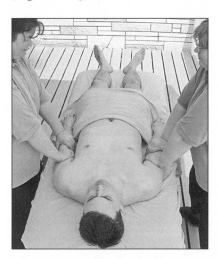

Figure A-19.2. *Synchronized palming up upper extremity*

Glide back down to fingertips with synchronized apana vayu stroke.
(Figure A-19.3)

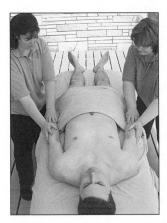

Figure A-19.3. *Synchronized apana vayu stroke*

Step 20. Neck and Feet

20. ASYNCHRONOUS—T1 NECK WORK, T2 FOOT WORK

T1—Sit at head of table. Time your first stroke with T2's first stroke.
Begin by stroking from shoulders to base of neck to base of skull. Lift
head to bring long hair forward to clear neck area. Apply oil to neck
and upper trapezius. Stroke from the base of the neck to the occiput
using both hands in an alternating fashion. Position fingers on occiput
and stretch neck gently by leaning your body weight backward. (Figure
A-20.1) Glide hands softly up back of head and slide off at the top.

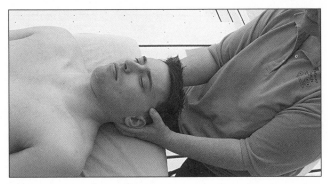

Figure A-20.1. Neck stretch

If the neck stretch causes pain, be careful not to perform additional stretches and deep tissue unless you are specifically trained in neck injury treatment. Advise client to seek professional medical attention. Position hands on the upper trapezius with fingers up. Use thumbs in circular pattern to loosen upper back muscles. (Figure A-20.2) Move laterally and back medially. Turn hands over and slide hands across shoulders, down upper arms, back up to neck, and back to base of skull.

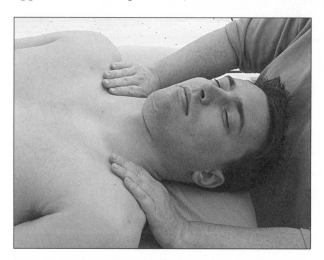

Figure A-20.2. Loosening upper back muscles

Carefully lift client's head and move to the left. Position your right hand on the right side of client's head and cross arms to place your left hand on client's shoulder. (Figure A-20.3) Gently move hands apart to stretch right neck muscles.

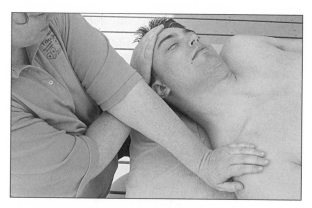

Figure A-20.3. Right neck stretch

Reposition left hand on client's forehead to stabilize head to side. With right hand in a loose fist and tucking thumb under fingers, slide your fist from lateral shoulder to base of neck, up neck to base of skull, and back down. (Figure A-20.4) Let your loose fingers conform to the contour of the client's body. Be careful to keep fingernails from touching skin. Rotate fist at base of neck several times. Slide up and down neck and out to shoulders, while rotating wrist to allow fingers to conform to the contours of the posterior neck and upper trapezius. Be careful to stay posterior to sternocleidomastoid to avoid putting any pressure on the carotid arteries. The carotid bifurcation at midneck is a common sight for plaque. If a piece of plaque breaks loose, the embolus could cause a stroke or transient ischemic attack.

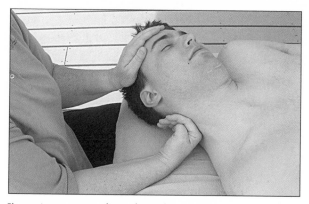

Figure A-20.4. Loose fist right neck massage

Reposition head to center. Perform a connecting effleurage stroke down neck, out to shoulders, back to neck, and up to base of skull. Carefully lift client's head and move to right. Position your left hand on the left side of client's head and cross arms to place your right hand on client's left shoulder. (Figure A-20.5) Gently move hands apart to stretch left neck muscles.

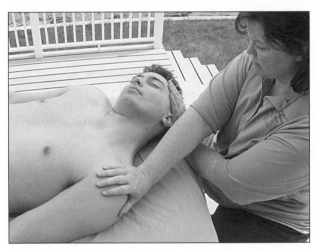

Figure A-20.5. Left neck stretch

Keep client's head to right side and reposition your right hand to client's forehead to stabilize head. With your left hand in a loose fist, tuck thumb under fingers, and slide your fist from lateral shoulder to base of neck, up neck to base of skull, and back down. (Figure A-20.6) Let your loose fingers conform to the contour of the client's body, while keeping fingernails away from skin. Rotate fist at base of neck several times. Slide up and down neck and out to shoulders, while rotating wrist to allow fingers to conform to the posterior neck and upper trapezius. Be careful to stay posterior to sternocleidomastoid to avoid the carotid arteries.

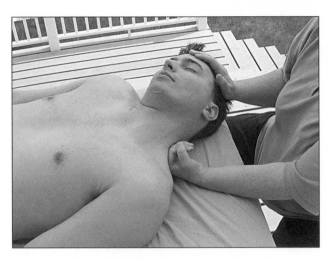

Figure A-20.6. Loose fist left neck massage

Bring head back to center. Perform another connecting effleurage stroke from base of skull to base of neck, out to shoulders, down arms, and back to base of skull. Lean backward to stretch neck again. Glide hands down back of neck. Slide your hands palm up under upper back. First, use a soothing, circular motion with hands on mid-upper back. Then feel the medial border of the scapula. Brace your middle and ring fingers with your other fingers and press up, leaving knuckles on bed for leverage. (Figure A-20.7) Alternatively, try turning wrist slightly and using the radial side of your index finger to exert the pressure. Use your other three fingers to support your index finger. Begin as close to the inferior angle of the scapula as you can. Slowly glide up edge of scapula. Stop at areas of tension and wait for a softening. You will feel the insertion of rhomboid major, rhomboid minor, and then levator scapulae. (Figure A-20.8)

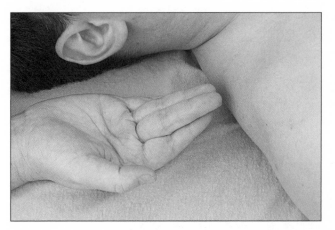

Figure A-20.7. Finger position to work insertion sites on medial scapula

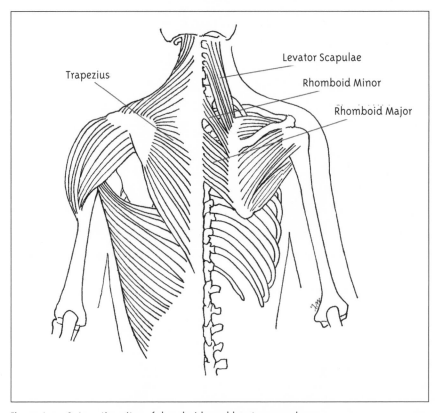

Figure A-20.8. Insertion sites of rhomboids and levator scapulae

Stop at the superior angle of the scapula, where you will likely feel tension. This is the insertion site of the levator scapulae. Wait for a release. Slowly work your way up the levator scapulae. Try to stay on course. The mid-section of the levator lies underneath the upper trapezius, so you will need to focus your pressure to get to the levator scapulae. This mid-section generally causes the most pain. Maintain deep pressure, but stop moving. Allow the muscle to melt and slide under your fingers on its own. Continue extremely slowly to the origin at the transverse processes of the top three or four vertebrae. (Figure A-20.9) If the levator scapulae are tight and/or tender, try a lesser pressure and repeat several times.

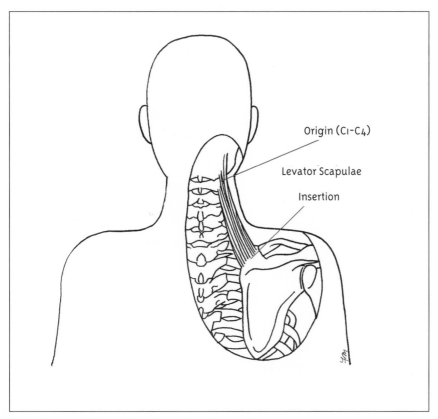

Figure A-20.9. Origin and insertion of levator scapulae

Soothe with circular strokes at the base of skull, down the neck, and the upper back. Slide hands to the top of shoulders. Push inferiorly with the right hand, then the left hand. Alternate downward pressure in a teeter-totter manner. (Figure A-20.10) This will help the levator scapulae to relax and lengthen.

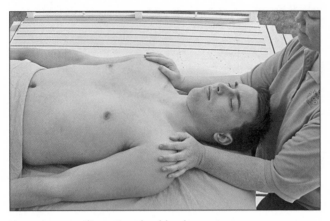

Figure A-20.10. Alternating shoulder depression

Stroke down arms and back to the shoulders. Glide palms of hands medially along the upper trapezius. Mobilize upper trapezius using heel of hand or soft thumb on bottom and flat fingers on top. (Figure A-20.11)

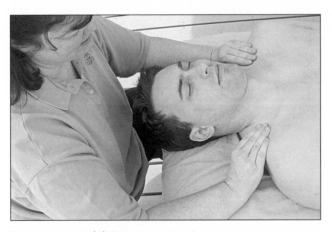

Figure A-20.11. Mobilizing upper trapezius

Stroke down the arms and back to the shoulders. Using flat palms, follow the clavicles to mid-anterior chest. Avoid the throat area. Soothe upper pectoral muscles with small circular pattern. Support your thumb with a closed fist and glide along inferior border of the clavicle from the sternum to shoulder. This will address the subclavius muscle and attachments of the pectoralis major. (Figure A-20.12) The subclavius courses beneath the pectoralis major. (Figure A-20.13) A shortened subclavius muscle may cause or contribute to pain in biceps and forearm and/or thoracic outlet syndrome (Davies 2004, p. 138). If tolerable to the client, you may wish to abduct and laterally rotate the humerus to provide a stretch.

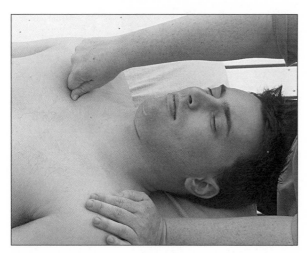

Figure A-20.12. Deep stroke below clavicle

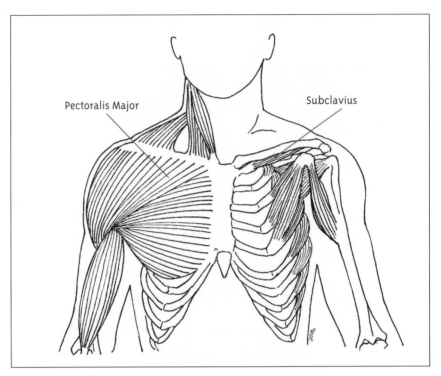

Figure A-20.13. Subclavius courses beneath pectoralis major

Slide back to sternum. Soothe areas above and below clavicle with effleurage. Hold client's head with your left hand and move your right forefinger and middle finger to the superior edge of clavicle. Lift client's head off table slightly, while moving it to opposite side. Feel for constrictions in the sternocleidomastoid and scalene attachments, while gently moving head in a manner that stretches that particular muscle (Riggs 2002, p. 129). Press in at areas of constriction and work the attachment site in both directions. (Figure A-20.14) Shortened scalene muscles refer pain to upper back, chest, shoulder, arm, and hand, which can lead to thoracic outlet syndrome and misdiagnoses of shortened rhomboids, muscle strains, tendinitis, and angina (Davies 2004, p. 80). Labored breathing, carrying heavy loads, and a forward head position are common causes of chronic hypertense scalene muscles (Davies 2004, p. 81). Repeat on the left side, while cradling head with your right hand.

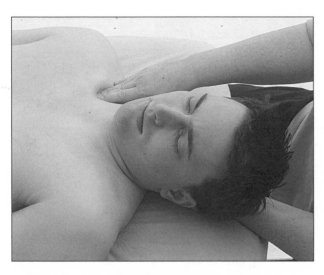

Figure A-20.14. Deep tissue above clavicle

Soothe with flat palm strokes. Effleurage down the arms, back up to the shoulders, and underneath the upper back. Soothe posterior neck muscles with effleurage by crossing index fingers at base of skull, sliding out laterally, moving toward base of neck, and repeating. Perform additional deep tissue massage of neck as your training permits. Deep neck massage is complex and requires hands-on training. When finished with deep tissue, reach as far down the spine as you can. Place supported middle and ring fingers on either side of the spine. Lift overlapped fingers slightly to create moderate pressure. Lean body weight backward as you glide your hands up the spine and neck to the base of the skull. (Figure A-20.15) Try not to lose contact. Gently pull at occiput for neck stretch. (Figure A-20.16)

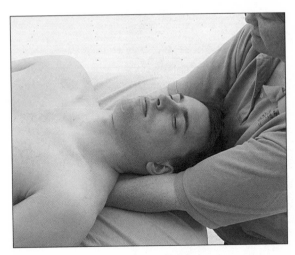

Figure A-20.15. Position for spinal glide

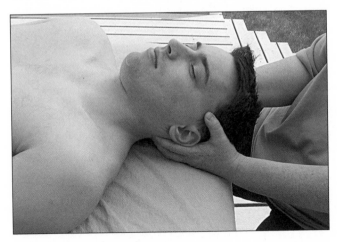

Figure A-20.16. Neck stretch

Without moving fingers, release pressure. Keep fingers and wrists straight and move hands in small circular pattern by moving elbows slightly and rocking forward and back with your upper body. (Figure A-20.17) This will relax the suboccipital muscles.

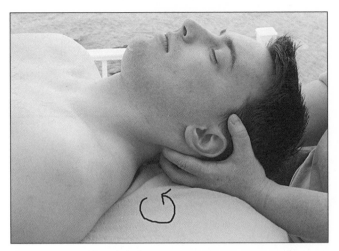

Figure A-20.17. Suboccipital massage

Slide hands to posterior head. Keep moving hands in circular pattern while rocking back and forth. (Figure A-20.18)

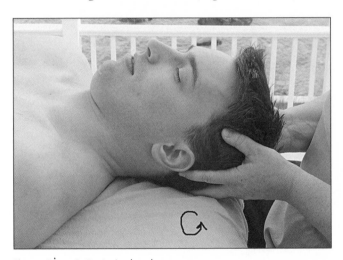

Figure A-20.18. Posterior head massage

Slide fingertips to top of head and keep massaging in small circular pattern. (Figure A-20.19)

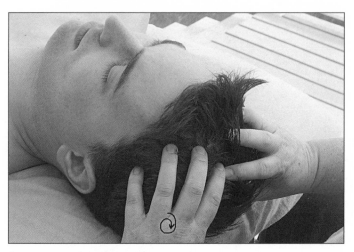

Figure A-20.19. Crown massage

Move hands to forehead with flat fingertips meeting in center of forehead. Move hands in small circular pattern. Move forehead skin without friction. (Figure A-20.20)

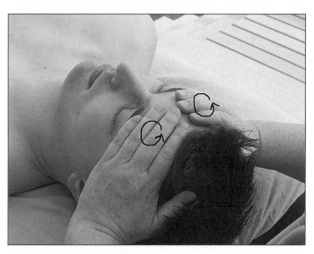

Figure A-20.20. Forehead massage

Slowly glide out to temporal region. Use very light pressure here. Move fingertips in circular pattern with no friction. (Figure A-20.21)

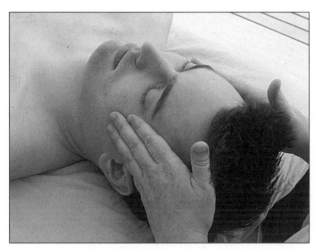

Figure A-20.21. Temporal massage

Slide down to masseter muscles. Cover entire masseter muscles with the palms of your hands. Wait momentarily to warm muscle. Move palms in circular pattern without friction. (Figure A-20.22)

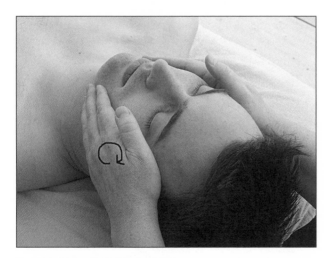

Figure A-20.22. Masseter massage

Press in with pads of fingertips along the mandible. This is the insertion of the masseter. Glide with medium pressure up to the origin of the masseter on the zygomatic arch (cheekbone). Glide back down the masseter to jaw and back up to cheek. Place pads of your index and middle fingers on anterior cheek and glide with medium pressure out laterally along the zygomatic arch to ear. This will address the origin of the masseter and the insertion of the temporalis. Repeat. (Figure A-20.23)

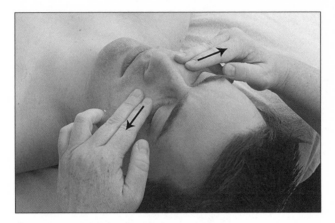

Figure A-20.23. Origin of masseter massage

Slide ulnar surface of hands along jawline, crossing at chin. (Figure A-20.24)

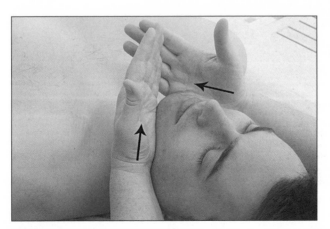

Figure A-20.24. Crossed hands at chin

With pads of fingertips, trace jawline back to temporomandibular joint. Gently slide underneath earlobes. Lightly grasp earlobes between thumb and forefinger. (Figure A-20.25) Massage entire external ear.

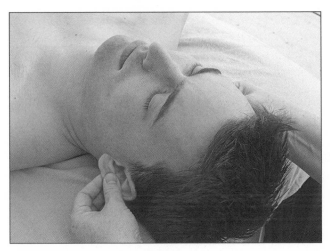

Figure A-20.25. External ear massage

Finish by pulling earlobes downward slightly and slide off. (Figure A-20.26)

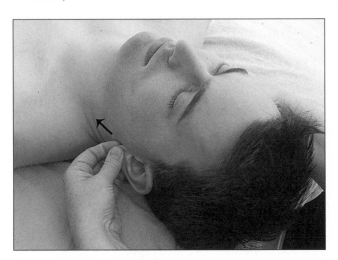

Figure A-20.26. Earlobe pull

Follow jawline back to chin. Place pad of thumbs in the center of chin just below the bottom lip. Spread tissue outward. (Figure A-20.27)

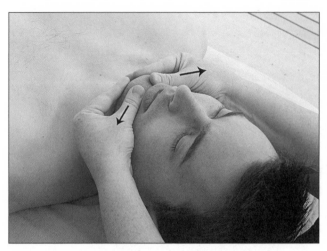

Figure A-20.27. Chin massage

Place thumbs just below nostrils. Glide out laterally. (Figure A-20.28)

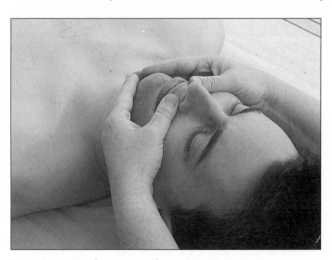

Figure A-20.28. Below nose stroke

Place thumbs near nose on zygomatic arch. Glide out laterally. (Figure A-20.29)

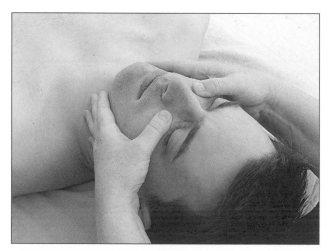

Figure A-20.29. Zygomatic arch stroke

Reposition pads of thumbs between eyebrows. Glide out laterally long eyebrows. (Figure A-20.30)

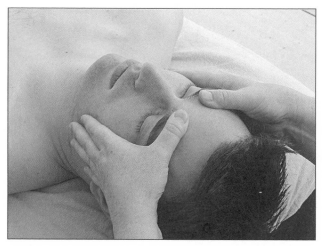

Figure A-20.30. Eyebrow stroke

Follow jawline again with ulnar surface of hands to cross at the chin. (Figure A-20.31)

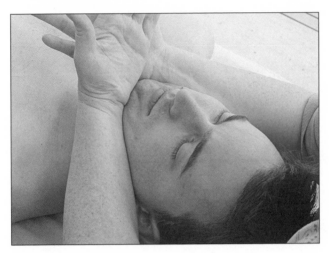

Figure A-20.31. Crossed hands at chin

Position flat hands gently on the face. Hold for a few moments. Silently ask for healing for your client. (Figure A-20.32)

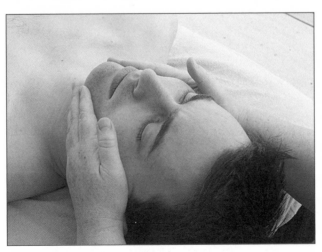

Figure A-20.32. Prayer for healing

Slide hands softly to the top of head and fall off at the end of the hair. (Figure A-20.33)

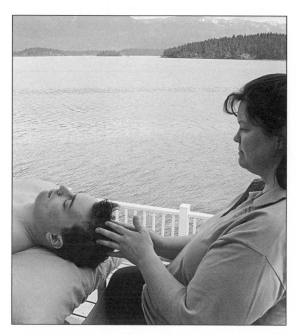

Figure A-20.33. Sliding off crown

T2—Sit at the foot of the table. Time your first stroke with T1's first stroke. Begin by stroking on top of sheet from mid-shin to tips of toes. Uncover one foot. Spread lotion from dorsum of foot up to mid-shin to follow direction of yin meridians. Wrap around to the posterior calf and glide down to ankle to follow the yang meridians. Repeat twice. Proceed over the ankle with one hand on top of the foot and one hand on bottom of foot to spread lotion over entire foot and toes. (Figure A-20.34)

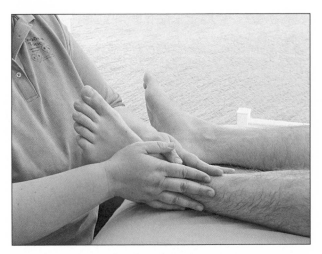

Figure A-20.34. Spreading lotion over foot

Petrissage lower calf and shin in an alternating handshake fashion. (Figure A-20.35)

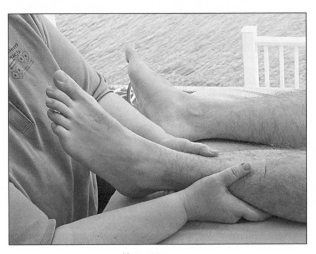

Figure A-20.35. Lower calf petrissage

With one hand on dorsum of foot and the other on bottom of foot, press hands gently together and rotate in a bicycle fashion. Move slowly to soothe entire foot and ankle. (Figure A-20.36)

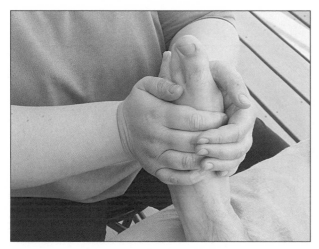

Figure A-20.36. Soothing entire foot

Perform deeper petrissage on anterior ankle and lower tibia. Use linear strokes from across ankle to lower shin. (Figure A-20.37)

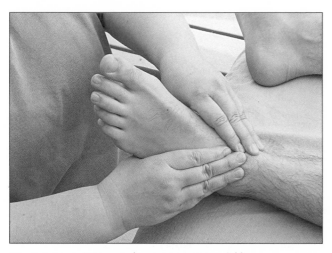

Figure A-20.37. Linear strokes across anterior ankle

Place hands on the medial and lateral sides of the ball of the foot. Move hands alternately forward and backward while moving hands to heel. (Figure A-20.38)

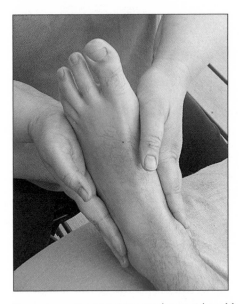

Figure A-20.38. Loosening muscles on sides of foot

Move hands to top and bottom of foot. Move hands alternately from side to side while moving to heel of foot. (Figure A-20.39)

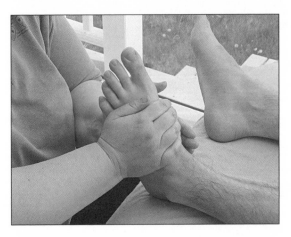

Figure A-20.39. Loosening top and bottom of foot

With the heels of your hands, hook into the area just above the ankle and jostle gently. Move inferior to ankle and jostle gently again. (Figure A-20.40)

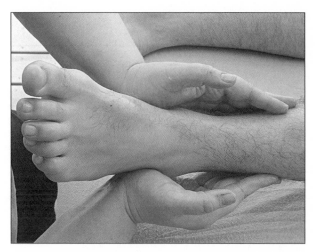

Figure A-20.40. Jostle ankle joint

Massage Achilles tendon with fingertips on either side. (Figure A-20.41) Continue massaging around to top of ankle in small circles.

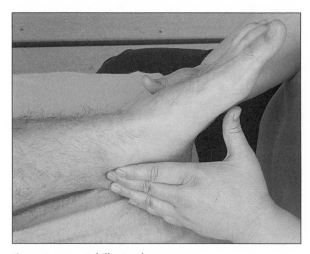

Figure A-20.41. Achilles tendon massage

Place thumbs on trigger point of the flexor digitorum brevis, just above the heel at bottom of arch. (Figure A-20.42) These trigger points refer pain to the ball of the foot and can add to plantar fasciitis. Press in with medium pressure. Hold thumbs steady while wrapping your fingers around to the top to the ankle. (Figure A-20.43) Glide fingertips in a transverse motion along the top of ankle while using thumbs on heel trigger points to flex and extend ankle. This will relax the ankle retinaculum to increase ankle flexibility. (Figure A-20.44)

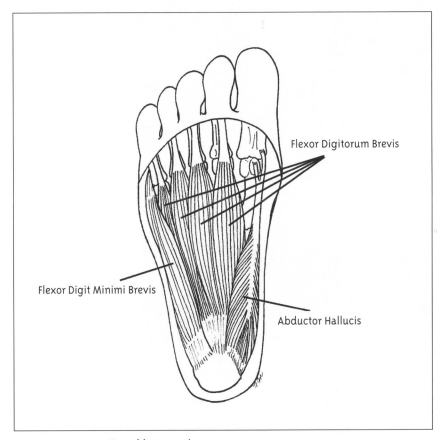

Figure A-20.42. Location of foot muscles

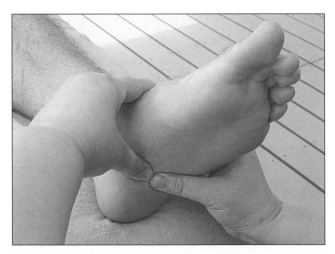

Figure A-20.43. Thumbs on trigger points of flexor digitorum brevis muscle

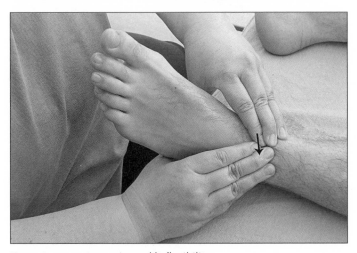

Figure A-20.44. Increasing ankle flexibility

Glide to toes. Bring thumbs to overlap at center of the top of the arch, just below the metatarsal heads and fingertips to overlap at center of top of foot. Squeeze in gently and slide out to sides of foot. This will create space between the metatarsals. Move toward toes and repeat until reaching the base of the toes. Spread base of toes in similar fashion. (Figure A-20.45)

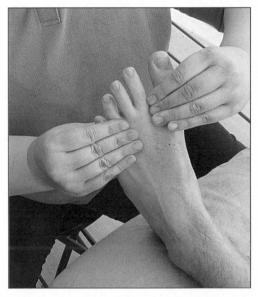

Figure A-20.45. Creating space between metatarsals

Soothe entire foot as in Figure A-20.36. Using a linear stroke with fingertips, glide between each metatarsal from base of toe to approximately half way up foot to the tarsal bones. (Figure A-20.46)

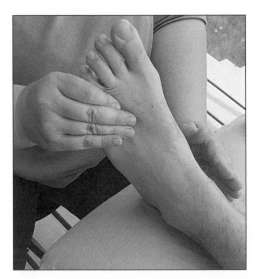

Figure A-20.46. Muscle massage between metatarsals

Concentrating on both the top and bottom of foot, begin with thumb at bottom of heel with fingertips on top of the ankle. Glide from the ankle to the tip of the toe along each metatarsal (not in-between). (Figure A-20.47) Stretch and rotate each toe at the end of each stroke. (Figure A-20.48)

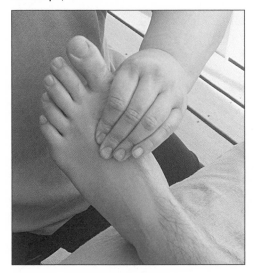

Figure A-20.47. Metatarsal glide

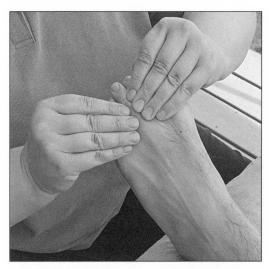

Figure A-20.48. Toe massage

Place your hand in a loosely closed fist. Line your knuckles up with the base of toes on the sole of the foot. Use your right hand for the right foot and your left hand for the left foot. Support the top of foot with your other hand. Push knuckles in and rotate down lateral (outside) edge of foot. Repeat. (Figure A-20.49)

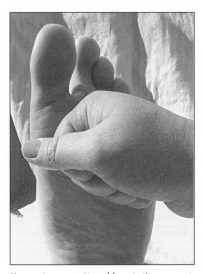

Figure A-20.49. Knuckle rotation on outer edge of sole of foot

Repeat soothing strokes over the entire foot and lower leg. Cover foot with sheet. Repeat all steps on opposite foot. When finished with both feet, brush downward from the knee (or as close to knee as you can reach) to the toes to bring any negative energy out. Place hands gently on ankles and perform healing energy until T1 finishes the head. (Figure A-20.50)

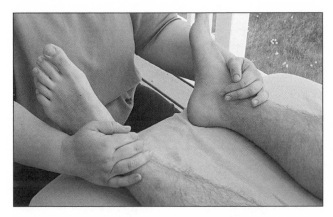

Figure A-20.50. Healing energy to finish foot sequence

T2—When T1 finishes head massage, grasp both posterior ankles.

T1—When you see that T2 is ready, place fingers along occiput on both sides.

Both therapists lean backward to create a stretch. (Figure A-20.51)

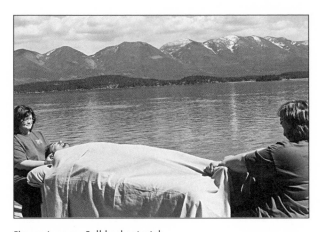

Figure A-20.51. Full body stretch

Step 21. Massage Completion

21. *SYNCHRONOUS—SEQUENCE TO COMPLETE MASSAGE*

T1 and T2 move to the head of the table. Place tips of fingers on either side of the top of the head and brush down both sides of the body simultaneously from head to toe. (Figure A-21.1) This movement is done with light pressure and relatively quick speed. Silently say, "Mind" or "Father." Repeat the stroke thinking, "Body" or "Son." Repeat once more thinking, "Spirit" or "Holy Spirit."

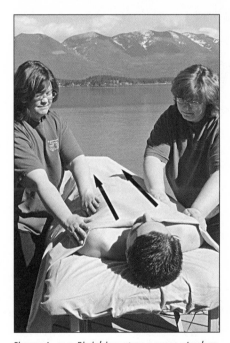

Figure A-21.1. *Finishing apana vayu strokes*

B. Sample Fifteen-Minute Seated Tandem Massage Routine
(Combination of shiatsu, trigger point, and Swedish)

Seated massage is a simple way to introduce clients to the concept of tandem massage without the intimidation of a full-hour table massage. This sample seated massage routine combines trigger point techniques with shiatsu and Swedish strokes to effectively release tension and free repetitive motion constrictions. It is the perfect antidote to stress at the workplace.

Pictures for the seated routine were taken at the beautiful KOA Campground in Polson, Montana.

Note: "Simultaneous" means that the therapists are performing similar, but not identical, strokes at the same time. "Synchronous" means that the therapists perform identical movements on either side of body at the same time. "Asynchronous" means that the movements of each therapist are not choreographed to match the other therapist, but are performed at same time. *Synchronous and simultaneous strokes are shown in italics,* while the asynchronous movements are shown in plain text.

1. *SIMULTANEOUS—BEGINNING STROKE*

T1—Stand behind the client and position fingertips on either side of the spine at base of neck.

T2—Stand facing the client and places fingertips on top of client's shoulders.

T1 and T2—Glide fingertips downward simultaneously. T1 glides from base of neck to sacrum. T2 glides from shoulders to fingertips.

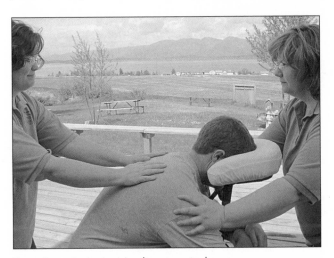

Figure B-1.1. *Beginning simultaneous stroke*

2. *SIMULTANEOUS—T1 LOOSENS LOW BACK, T2 LOOSENS TRAPEZIUS*

T1—Place the heel of your left hand on the client's left hip (PSIS) and the heel of your right hand on the client's right hip (PSIS). (Figure B-2.1) Slowly lean your body weight into your left hand. Compress in and down. Hold momentarily and release. Shift your weight to your right hand. Compress in and down. Hold momentarily and release. Repeat process numerous times to create a gentle rolling sensation to loosen low back and hips.

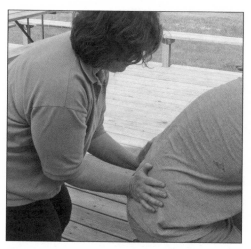

Figure B-2.1. *Loosening lower back and hips*

T2—Position your hands on client's shoulders. (Figure B-2.2) Slowly lean your body weight downward onto the client's left shoulder. Roll the shoulder gently in a small circular fashion, directing pressure inferiorly, anteriorly, superiorly, and posteriorly. Release pressure on the left shoulder and repeat on right shoulder. Perform consecutively numerous times in a gentle rolling pattern to loosen and stretch the upper trapezius. This is a shiatsu movement called "cat paws."

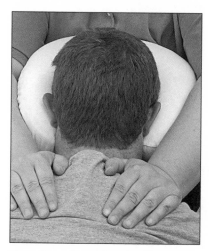

Figure B-2.2. *Loosening shoulders*

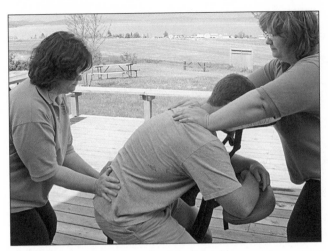

Figure B-2.3. *Loosening lower back and shoulders*

3. ASYNCHRONOUS—T1 PALMS DOWN BLADDER MERIDIAN, T2 PALMS DOWN BOTH ARMS

T1—Place heels of hands on either side of the upper thoracic spine. (Figure B-3.1) Allow palms to conform to body. Lean body weight into the heel of hands to create an even pressure. Hold the compression for several seconds and release. Move one palm-width down and repeat. T1 repeats this process until the sacrum is reached.

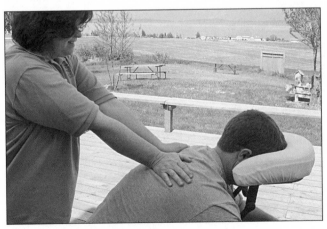

Figure B-3.1. Palming the bladder meridian

T2—Spread your thumbs and index fingers in "dragon's mouth" shape. Place left "dragon's mouth" on client's right shoulder and your right hand on client's left shoulder. (Figure B-3.2) Lean body weight forward and hold for several seconds. Release and move several inches toward hands and repeat to wrists.

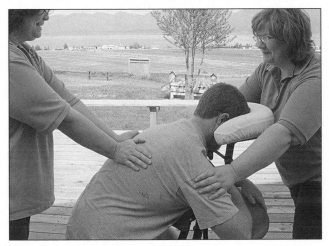

Figure B-3.2. "Dragon's mouth" on both arms

4. ASYNCHRONOUS—T1 THUMBS BLADDER MERIDIAN, T2 PALMS DOWN LEFT ARM

T1—Thumb down Bladder 1 meridian (Figure B-4.1) by placing pads of thumbs close to spine on either side. Lean body weight forward to create an even pressure with thumbs. Hold and release. Move thumbs down several thumb-widths and repeat to sacrum. (Figure B-4.2)

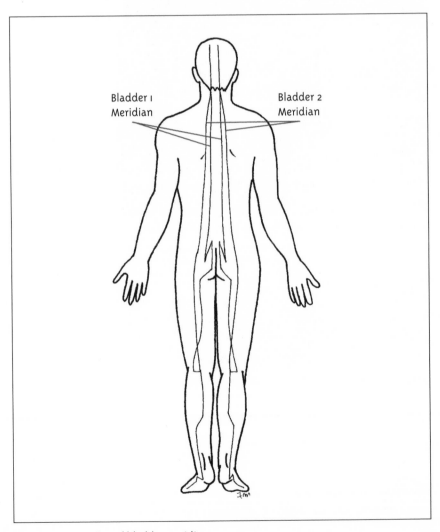

Figure B-4.1. Location of bladder meridians

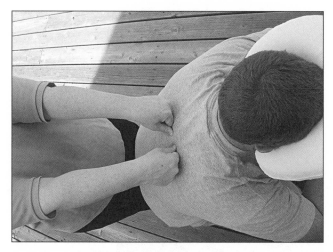

Figure B-4.2. Thumbing down Bladder 1 meridian

T2—Palm down from left shoulder to wrist. Begin by holding client's left wrist with your left hand. Spread your right thumb and index finger in "dragon's mouth" shape. Place "dragon's mouth" on client's left shoulder. (Figure B-4.3) Lean body weight forward and hold for several seconds. Release and move several inches toward hand and repeat to wrist.

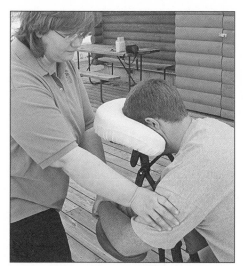

Figure B-4.3. "Dragon's mouth" on left arm

5. ASYNCHRONOUS—T1 THUMBS DOWN BLADDER 2 MERIDIAN, T2 STRETCHES LEFT HAND

T1—Thumb down Bladder 2 meridian by placing thumbs on lateral edge of erector spinae (an inch or so lateral to middle of spine). (Figure B-5.1)

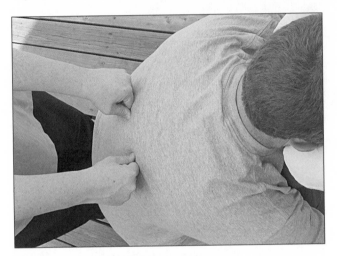

Figure B-5.1. Thumbing Bladder 2 meridian

Again, body weight is used to exert pressure and then thumbs are moved inferiorly to repeat pressure. From the bottom of ribcage to the top of the iliac crest, pressure is directed at oblique angle (medially toward spine and anteriorly toward front of client) to avoid putting any pressure directly into the kidneys. (Figure B-5.2)

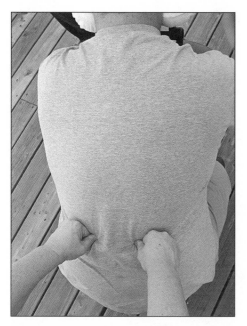

Figure B-5.2. Oblique angle thumbing

T2—Begin work on left wrist and hand by placing hands on either side of client's left wrist. Jostle gently to mobilize wrist joint. Rotate wrist in bicycle fashion. (Figure B-5.3)

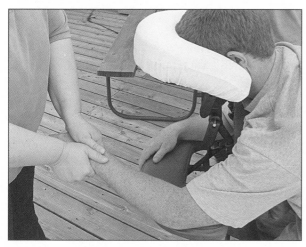

Figure B-5.3. Left wrist mobilization

Slide hands out to first knuckles of client's hand. Support his hand with the fingers of both of your hands. Place your thumbs between each large knuckle at the metacarpophalangeal joint. Apply pressure and stroke down toward wrist between each metacarpal to the carpal bones. (Figure B-5.4) Pay particular attention to the thumb metacarpal.

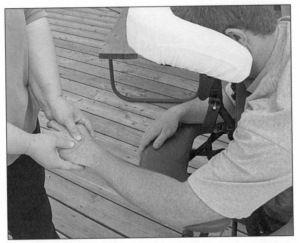

Figure B-5.4. Linear strokes on dorsum of hand

Invert the client's hand, so his palm is facing up. Place your little finger between the client's index and middle fingers. Place the little finger of your other hand between the client's ring and little fingers. Support your client's hand with your other fingers. (Figure B-5.5) Move your little fingers gently apart to stretch the client's hand.

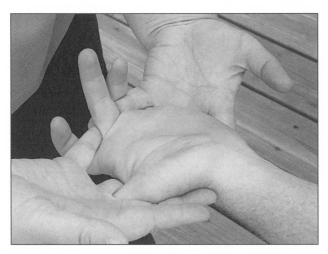

Figure B-5.5. Left hand stretch

Press in at the center of the heel of the client's palm with both thumbs. Glide to sides of hand to stretch palm muscles. Move toward fingers and repeat. Repeat to knuckles and back to the heel of hand. (Figure B-5.6)

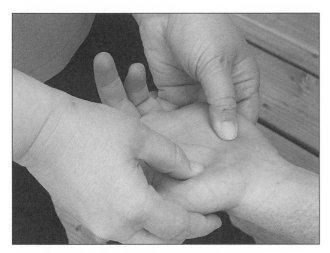

Figure B-5.6. Gliding and stretching palm muscles

6. ASYNCHRONOUS—T1 RELEASES TRIGGER POINTS OF LEFT SHOULDER AREA, T2 COMPLETES LEFT HAND-MASSAGE

T1—Locate trigger points on and around left shoulder by feeling for any knots or constrictions with relaxing petrissage. Common trigger points occur at the medial border of scapula, superior angle of the scapula, and along the spine of the scapula. (Figure B-6.1) Ask the client if a potential trigger point is tender and if pain refers. Press the trigger or tender point with either one thumb on top of the other or the point of your elbow. (Figure B-6.2) Ask client to tell you when pain subsides. If the pain does not subside in reasonable amount of time, you may need to move slightly to hit the spot. Usually, the actual site will release relatively quickly. Release and soothe with light petrissage. Locate the next trigger point. Repeat as necessary. A trigger point tool is helpful to prevent injury to thumbs.

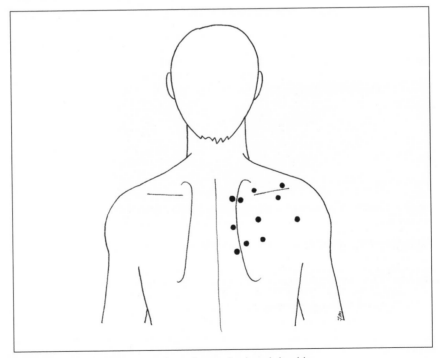

Figure B-6.1. Common trigger points of upper back and shoulders

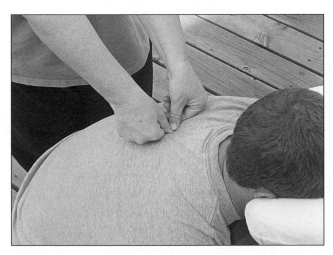

Figure B-6.2. Trigger point compression

T2—Release stretch by removing your little fingers. Turn client's hand palm down. Grasp client's thumb between your index and middle fingers. Pull gently to create space in the joints. (Figure B-6.3) Release and reposition thumb between your thumb and forefinger to massage from first knuckle and slide off at tip. Repeat with each finger.

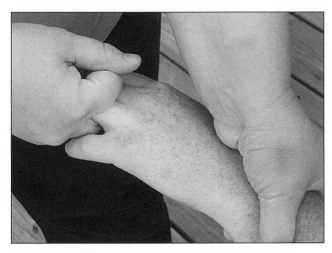

Figure B-6.3. Pulling digits to create space in left hand joints

7. SYNCHRONOUS—ARM STROKE

T1 moves to the left shoulder and T2 moves to the right side to position hands on the right shoulder.

T1 and T2 simultaneously stroke down from shoulder to fingertips. (Figure B-7.1)

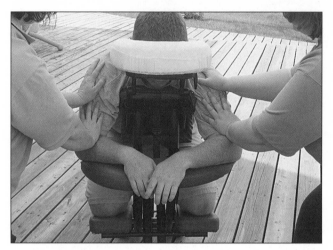

Figure B-7.1. *Synchronous arm stroke*

8. SYNCHRONOUS—ARM STRETCH

T1—Use your left hand to lift client's left arm to a ninety-degree angle. Interlock your right elbow with client's left elbow.

T2—Use your right hand to lift client's right arm to a ninety-degree angle. Interlock your left elbow with client's right elbow.

T1, T2—Shift body weight backward to stretch upper arm and shoulder girdle. This passive shiatsu stretch is called "crane's embrace." (Figure B-8.1)

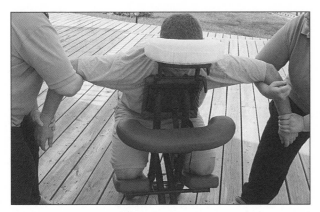

Figure B-8.1. *Tandem "crane's embrace"*

9. SIMULTANEOUS—T1 STRETCHES LEFT ANTERIOR SHOULDER, T2 STRETCHES RIGHT POSTERIOR SHOULDER

T1—Swing client's left arm back and forth, then place his left hand on the top of his head. Slowly stretch the client's elbow backward with your left hand. Place your right mother hand on the medial border of the left scapula. (Figure B-9.1) Repeat the stretch several times.

T2—Grasp the client's right wrist and gently pull his arm forward. Lean your body weight backward slowly to create an even stretch of the posterior shoulder. (Figure B-9.1)

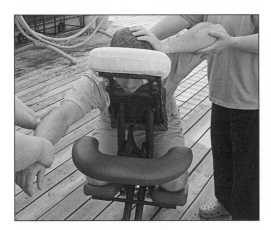

Figure B-9.1. *Left anterior shoulder and right posterior shoulder stretch*

10. ASYNCHRONOUS—T1 LOOSENS LEFT SHOULDER, T2 PALMS DOWN
   RIGHT ARM

T1—Swing client's left arm back and forth and position behind his back. Use your left forearm to ease the shoulder and arm backward. Use the radial aspect of your right hand or fingertips to press deeply under the shoulder blade, while pulling shoulder back with your left forearm. (Figure B-10.1)

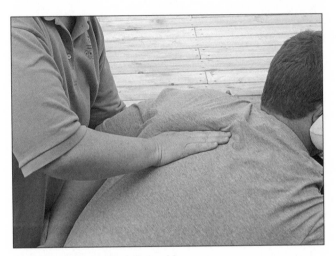

Figure B-10.1. Loosening left shoulder

T2—Return client's right arm to armrest, palm down from right shoulder to wrist. Begin by holding client's right wrist with your right hand. Spread your left thumb and index finger in the "dragon's mouth" shape. Place "dragon's mouth" on the client's right shoulder. Lean body weight forward and hold for several seconds. Release and move several inches toward the hand and repeat to the wrist. (Figure B-10.2)

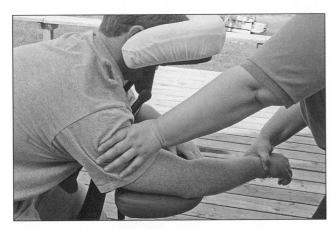

Figure B-10.2. "Dragon's mouth" on right arm

11. ASYNCHRONOUS—T1 RELEASES TRIGGER POINTS OF RIGHT SHOULDER AREA, T2 MASSAGES RIGHT HAND

T1—Locate trigger points on and around right shoulder and upper back. (Figure B-6.1) Feel for constrictions or knots. Ask the client if a potential trigger point is tender and if pain refers. Press the trigger point with either one thumb on top of the other or the point of your elbow. (Figure B-11.1) Hold until pain subsides. Repeat as necessary.

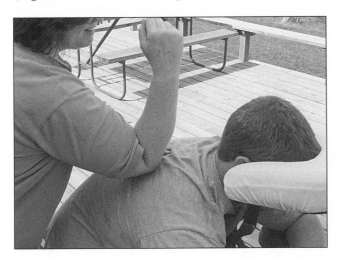

Figure B-11.1. Right shoulder and upper back trigger point release

T2—Begin work on right wrist and hand by placing hands on either side of client's right wrist with palm of hand down. Jostle gently to mobilize wrist joint. Rotate wrist in bicycle fashion. (Figure B-11.2)

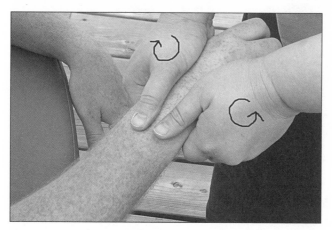

Figure B-11.2. Right wrist mobilization

Slide hands out to the first knuckles of the client's hand. Support his hand with the fingers of both of your hands. Place your thumbs between each large knuckle at the metacarpophalangeal joint. Apply pressure and stroke down toward wrist between each metacarpal to the carpal bones. (Figure B-11.3) Pay particular attention to the thumb metacarpal.

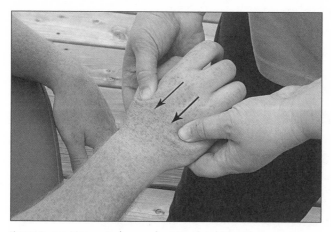

Figure B-11.3. Linear strokes on dorsum of right hand

Invert the client's hand, so palm is facing up. Place your little finger between the client's index and middle fingers. Place the little finger of your other hand between the client's ring and little fingers. Support the client's hand with your other fingers. (Figure B-11.4) Move your little fingers gently apart to stretch the client's hand.

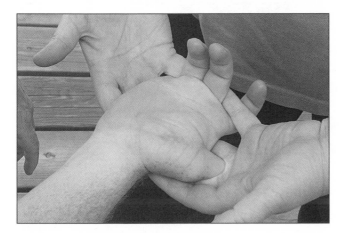

Figure B-11.4. Right hand stretch

Press in at the center of the heel of client's palm with both thumbs. Glide to sides of the hand to stretch palm muscles. Move toward the fingers and repeat. Repeat to knuckles and back to the heel of hand. (Figure B-11.5)

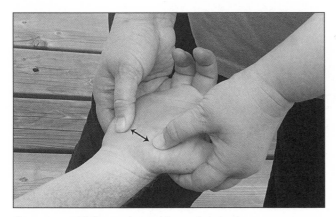

Figure B-11.5. Gliding and stretching palm muscles

Release stretch by removing your little fingers. Turn client's hand palm down. Grasp client's thumb between your index and middle fingers. Pull gently to create space in the joints. (Figure B-11.6) Release and massage to slide off at tip. Repeat with each finger.

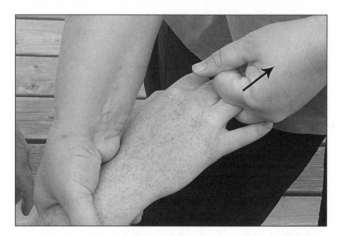

Figure B-11.6. Pulling digits to create space in joints

12. SYNCHRONOUS—ARM STROKE

T1 and T2 simultaneously stroke down from shoulder to fingertips, T1 on right and T2 on left. (Figure B-12.1)

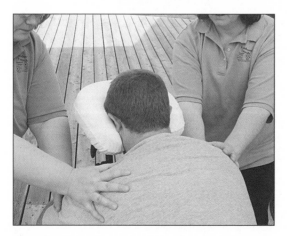

Figure B-12.1. *Synchronous arm stroke*

13. SIMULTANEOUS—T1 STRETCHES RIGHT ANTERIOR SHOULDER, T2 STRETCHES LEFT POSTERIOR SHOULDER

T1—Swing client's right arm back and forth, then place his right hand on top of his head. Slowly stretch client's elbow backward with your right hand. Place your left hand ("mother hand") on the medial border of the right scapula. Repeat the stretch several times. (Figure B-13.1)

T2—Grasp the client's left wrist and pull his arm straight forward. Lean your body weight slowly backward to create an even stretch of the posterior shoulder. (Figure B-13.1)

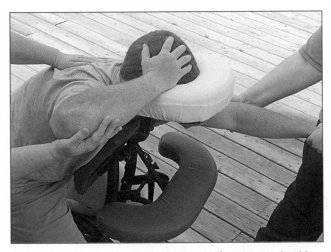

Figure B-13.1. *Right anterior shoulder and left posterior shoulder stretch*

14. ASYNCHRONOUS—T1 LOOSENS RIGHT SHOULDER, T2 COMPRESSES "THREE PEARLS"

T1—Swing the client's right arm back and forth and position behind his back. Use your right forearm to ease your client's shoulder and arm backward. Use the radial aspect of your left hand or fingertips to press deeply under the shoulder blade while pulling the shoulder back with forearm. (Figure B-14.1)

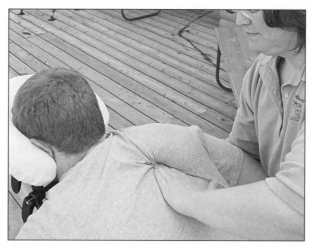

Figure B-14.1. Loosening right shoulder

T2—Place index, middle, and ring fingers of both hands along the client's occipital ridge ("three pearls"). (Figure B-14.2) Exert an upward, pulling pressure with left fingers. Hold pressure for several seconds and release. Repeat with right fingers. Perform consecutively several times to loosen and stretch the neck.

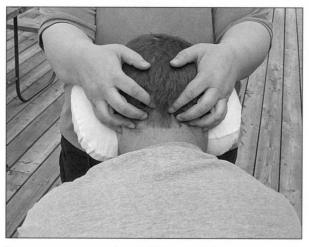

Figure B-14.2. Compressing the "three pearls"

15. ASYNCHRONOUS—T1 MASSAGES NECK, T2 MASSAGES SCALP

T1—With left hand at base of the neck and right hand at the top of neck at occipital ridge, knead neck muscles by pressing your thumb and fingers together. Alternate squeezing pressure from the left to the right hand in a smooth, slow rhythm of squeezing and releasing. (Figure B-15.1)

T2—Use small, circular strokes with fingertips beginning at the base of the neck. Reposition fingertips and repeat until entire scalp is massaged. (Figure B-15.1)

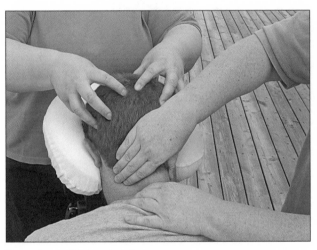

Figure B-15.1. Neck and scalp massage

16. SYNCHRONOUS—UPPER TRAPEZIUS STRETCH

T1 and T2—Grasp the upper trapezius muscle with fingertips. Bend your knees to direct body weight downward and outward for a slow stretch. (Figure B-16.1)

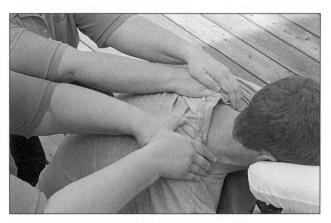

Figure B-16.1. *Bilateral trapezius stretch*

17. SYNCHRONOUS—BACK PETRISSAGE

T1 and T2—Begin at shoulders and work your way down back with rhythmical alternating open-C, closed-C strokes. Match your rhythm and pressure with your associate's. (Figure B-17.1)

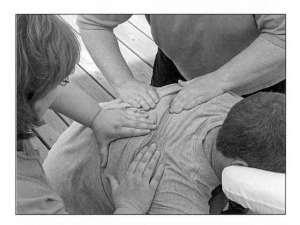

Figure B-17.1. *Synchronous back petrissage*

18. SYNCHRONOUS—BACK VIBRATION

T1 and T2—Bring both hands to top of shoulders. With fingertips, move hands quickly back and forth to create vibratory effect. Stroke downward from upper trapezius to iliac crest. Keep wrists and fingers straight. Move elbows to create short back and forth motion. Repeat three times. (Figure B-18.1)

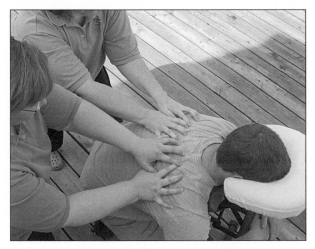

Figure B-18.1. *Synchronous back vibration*

19. SYNCHRONOUS—BACK PERCUSSION ("Hacking")

T1 and T2—Perform synchronous hacking. Begin at iliac crest and work your way up to the shoulders and back down to the iliac crest. With your wrists relaxed, use the ulnar surface of your hands and little finger in an alternating fashion to strike the body lightly and briskly. Keep your fingers relaxed and slightly apart to act as shock absorbers. Your fingers should knock together. Match your fellow therapist's strokes as well as you can in strength, speed, and location. (Figure B-19.1)

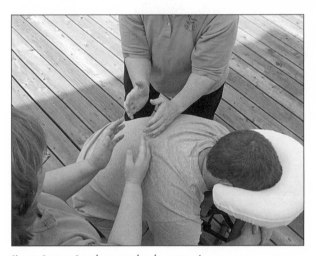

Figure B-19.1. *Synchronous back percussion*

20. FINISHING SIMULTANEOUS STROKE

T1—Stand behind the client and position fingertips on either side of the spine at the base of the neck.

T2—Promptly move to face the client and place fingertips on the client's shoulders.

T1 and T2—Glide fingertips downward simultaneously. T1 glides from the base of the neck to the sacrum. T2 glides from the shoulders to the fingertips, as in Step 1. This movement is done quickly and simultaneously to rejuvenate the client. Repeat three times, thinking mind-body-spirit. (Figure B-20.1)

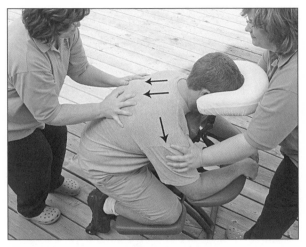

Figure B-20.1. *Simultaneous stroke to complete seated massage*

Tandem seated massage, fifteen dollars.
Happy and relaxed client, priceless! (Figure B-20.2)

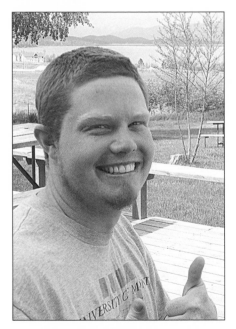

Figure B-20.2 Happy client

C. Sample Tandem Subroutine for Piriformis Syndrome
(Combination of deep tissue, trigger point, and Swedish)

This sample subroutine is provided to stimulate your creativity in using two therapists to generate more effective treatments and to illustrate how specific deep tissue techniques can be modified for tandem massage. Developing subroutines for the most common conditions that you see in your practice is extremely valuable. Subroutines can be readily inserted into your one-hour integrative massage routine.

All subroutines need not be as elaborate as this sample. You may simply need to modify your usual routine. For example, when additional neck work is needed, the order can be changed. When the client turns over to a supine position, the therapists could do the arms before the legs. The arms would be done as usual. After completing the arms, the first therapist could go straight to the neck. The second therapist would massage both left and right legs and feet, thus increasing therapist one's neck time. Variations like this make the massage very smooth, yet allow extra time for troublesome areas.

We gratefully acknowledge that several techniques in this subroutine were adapted from *Deep Tissue Massage: A Visual Guide to Techniques* by Art Riggs.

Insert the Subroutine for Piriformis Syndrome into the Tandem One-Hour Routine between steps three and four. You will likely need to subtract some of the deep tissue work in the asynchronous sections to make up the time difference. There are no synchronous movements in this subroutine.

1. IDENTIFY PIRIFORMIS AND OTHER TIGHT ROTATORS

After relaxing the lower back and gluteus muscles, begin by identifying the piriformis and other deep lateral hip rotators. (Figure C-1.1)

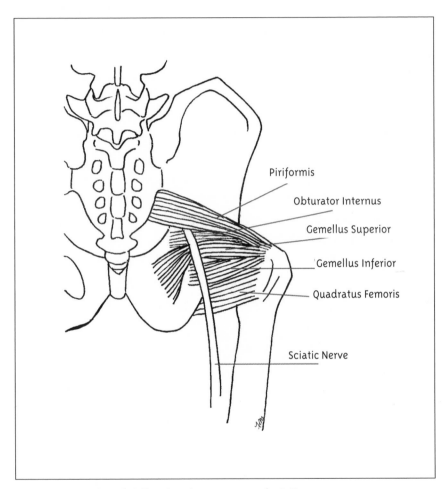

Piriformis

Obturator Internus

Gemellus Superior

Gemellus Inferior

Quadratus Femoris

Sciatic Nerve

Figure C-1.1. Location of piriformis, other rotators, and sciatic nerve

T1—Position your hands one on top of the other to support your fingers. Place your fingertips about one-half inch from the medial edge of the greater trochanter.

T2—Bend client's knee to a ninety-degree angle by holding the ankle. Slowly move client's lower leg out laterally, while the knee is kept on the table. This will flex the hip rotators. (Figure C-1.2)

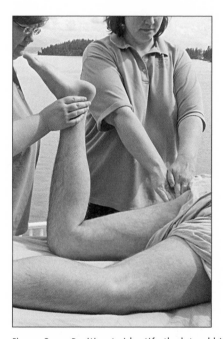

Figure C-1.2. Position to identify the lateral hip rotators

T1—Press in slowly to feel for movement.

T2—Swing the ankle gently back and forth approximately three to four inches and repeat until T1 identifies the piriformis and other rotators with certainty. (Figure C-1.3)

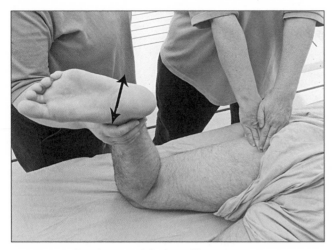

Figure C-1.3. Identification of the lateral hip rotators

2. MASSAGE INSERTION SITES OF THE ROTATORS AT THE GREATER TROCHANTER

T2—With the client's knee in a ninety-degree angle, hold the client's leg out laterally to put the rotators into a gentle stretch.

T1—Use supported fingertips to gently massage the insertion of the lateral hip rotators on the greater trochanter. (Figure C-2.1) The tip of your elbow would work as well. Move fingertips slowly, trying to feel the tight spots. Stop and maintain your pressure when you feel tightness. Wait for a release. Be sure to tell the client to breathe into the area and to tell you if he feels any numbness, tingling, or shooting pain. If these symptoms occur, then ease up on the pressure and/or change the angle at which you are applying pressure. Always use an oblique angle. Never angle straight down into the pelvis. You must guard against further sciatic nerve irritation.

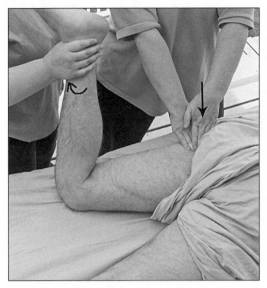

Figure C-2.1. Massaging insertions of lateral hip rotators

3. APPLY PRESSURE NEAR ORIGIN OF PIRIFORMIS

The piriformis originates on the anterior surface of the sacrum, near the halfway point.

T1—Take over holding the client's ankle. While T2 is moving to the other side of the table, jostle the leg gently to relax the muscles and reduce guarding. Then, hold your client's leg steady with his knee at a ninety-degree angle and with the calf laterally rotated to stretch the rotators again. If possible, hold the leg with your inferior hand and place your superior hand on the sacrum to anchor the tissue. You will need to point fingers inferiorly in order to allow room for your associate to work along the edge of the sacrum.

T2—Move to the opposite side of the table. Remove draping. Put one hand on top of the other to support your fingers. Locate the edge of the sacrum. Position your fingertips near the origin of the piriformis on the edge of the sacrum at the halfway point. Apply oblique pressure away from the sacrum toward the greater trochanter. Hold and wait for a release. (Figure C-3.1)

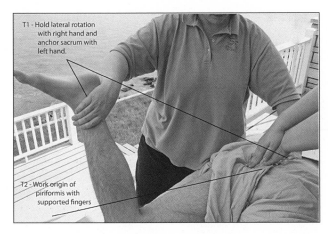

Figure C-3.1. Origin of piriformis work with sacrum anchor and stretch

4. WORK ORIGIN OF QUADRATUS FEMORIS

T1—Release the stretch and lay the client's leg back down on the table. Take a step closer to the head of the table. While T2 is coming back around the table, place the heel of your hand midway between the greater trochanter and ischial tuberosity and gently press in. Move the heel of your hand in a small, circular pattern. (Figure C-4.1) This will relax the hip rotators. Stop when T2 is in position.

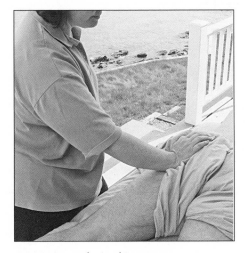

Figure C-4.1. Relaxing hip rotators

T2—Come back around the foot of the table and stand next to T1. Locate the greater trochanter and move medially to locate the ischial tuberosity (sitting bone). Using your knuckle, slowly sink in and make contact with the bone. This will affect the origin of the quadratus femoris (one of the other rotators) and have the added effect of relaxing the gluteals and insertion of the hamstrings. (Figure C-4.2)

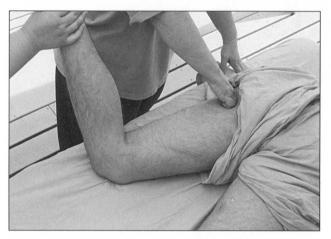

Figure C-4.2. Using knuckle at origin of quadratus femoris

5. CONTINUE WITH STEPS FOUR THROUGH TEN OF THE TANDEM ONE-HOUR ROUTINE

6. PERFORM AN EXTRA STRETCH ON AFFECTED LEG

During either step ten or step twelve of the tandem one-hour routine (depending on which is the affected leg), perform an additional piriformis stretch. This will be during the asynchronous section with the other leg stretched in supine position. Ask your client to cross the ankle of his affected leg over his other knee. Then, bring his knee (of his unaffected leg) up toward his shoulder. (Figure C-6.1)

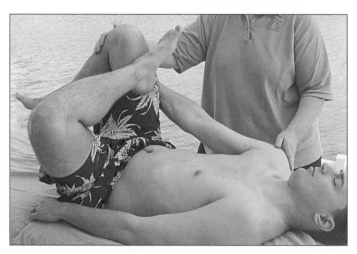

Figure C-6.1. Additional piriformis stretch

You may assist him. Make sure his sacrum remains on the table. Ask him to perform this stretch at home once a day and hold the stretch for thirty seconds.

7. FINISH THE REST OF THE ONE-HOUR TANDEM ROUTINE

References

Battle, Michael. *Reconciliation: The Ubuntu Theology of Desmond Tutu,* Cleveland, OH: The Pilgrim Press, 1997.

Chabot, Karyn. *Ayurvedic Mirror Massage,* Middletown, RI: Sacred Stone Center for Holistic Education and Therapy, 2002, www.sacredstonehealing.com

Davies, Clair. *The Trigger Point Therapy Workbook: Your Self-Treatment Guide for Pain Relief,* second edition, Oakland, CA: New Harbinger Publications, Inc., 2004.

Jarmey, Chris. *The Concise Book of Muscles,* Berkeley, CA: North Atlantic Books, 2003.

Johnson, Jim. *The Multifidus Back Pain Solution: Simple Exercises That Target the Muscles That Count,* Oakland, CA: New Harbinger Publications, Inc., 2002.

KOA Campground of Polson/Flathead Lake. Owners Paul and Carlisa London, Hwy. 93 North, Polson, MT 59860, www.polsonkoa.com, (406) 883-2151.

Merton, Thomas. "Haga Sophia," in *A Thomas Merton Reader,* ed. Thomas P. McDonnell, New York: Doubleday, 1989.

Northwest School of Massage. Director Jack Weaver, 720 South 333rd St., Ste. 101, Federal Way, WA 98003, www.nwsm.net, (800) 929-9441.

Parker, Palmer J. *Let Your Life Speak,* San Francisco, CA: Jossey-Bass, Inc., 2000.

Riggs, Art. *Deep Tissue Massage: A Visual Guide to Techniques,* Berkeley, CA: North Atlantic Books, 2002.

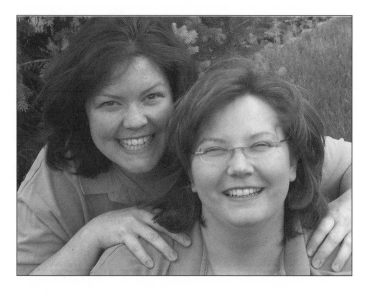

About the Authors

Terri and Tammi Tremper live in Polson, Montana, where they own
and operate Tandem Touch Therapeutic Massage. The twin sisters grad-
uated from the Northwest School of Massage in Federal Way,
Washington, and are nationally certified massage therapists and bodyworkers. In addition, they are educated in deep tissue, shiatsu, Swedish
massage, injury treatment, craniosacral therapy, Reiki, and Jin Shin Do.
The Trempers obtained additional certification in Ayurvedic Tandem
Mirror Massage through Sacred Stone Center for Holistic Education
in Rhode Island. They have since developed their own innovative
approach to tandem massage that incorporates contemporary therapeutic massage techniques into the ancient practice of Mirror Massage.